I0493367

The Essential U.S. Guide to Chemotherapy and Radiation:

What You Need to Know

Jennifer Reinoehl

Contents

Many thanks to Shirley C. and Briohne Sykes (Sneaky Happiness), who have been down this road, survived, and were willing to share with others about it. Special thanks to Larry and Bob P. who are still bravely walking the road. And to Scott B. and D. D. who not only are fighting through cancer but also the loss of immediate family members. Without their information and first hand accounts this book would not have been possible.

Also, thanks to Java Davis for making sure this book wasn't too technical.

Introduction

In 2011, around 1,530,000 people in the United States were newly diagnosed with cancer according to the National Cancer Institute. Cancer survival rates also have improved steadily over the period from 2001–2008. For example, the overall ten-year survival rate for testis cancer was almost 100% in 2007 (the last year for which data was collected) and breast cancer survival jumped from around 60% in 1991 to almost 80% in 2007. New methods of radiation therapy and chemotherapy and new technologies are being developed every day, which continue to boost long-term survival rates.

Radiation therapy and chemotherapy are used more frequently than many other treatments for cancer and tumors. However, few people know exactly what to expect from these treatments until they have gone through them. The uncertainty can cause unnecessary worry and distress. Adding to these fears are stories from the past when radiation and chemotherapy were in their early stages of development. Now, much has changed in the way these cancer-fighting tools are used so that patients have the fewest side effects with the most benefits.

You may be confused about these treatments by the many rumors and stories on the web, and you may need more information about them. Or perhaps you already have begun your treatments and have had a difficult time with side effects. Wherever you are on your road to being cancer-

"In 2011, around 1,530,000 people in the United States were newly diagnosed with cancer..."

free, this book will help you understand what you are going through so you can get back to your life.

This book was created for those who have been diagnosed with cancer and who have been told they need radiation and/or chemotherapy. It is also for the friends and loved ones of those undergoing these treatments. It was designed to further explain things you may have heard from your health care provider in terms that are easy to understand if are uncertain about them.

'Cancer strikes across age levels, but it is certainly not the death sentence that it once was.'

In *The Essential U.S. Guide to Chemotherapy and Radiation: What You Need to Know*, you will find the most up-to-date information on radiation and chemotherapy. This book will explain what these treatments are and how they affect cancer. It will discuss side effect you may have and ways to overcome them. There is an entire chapter devoted to friends and family to help them understand the treatments and ways they can assist their loved ones. Finally, it discusses how to best continue with your life once your treatments are complete.

For friends and family members, this book can help you to learn what is happening as your loved one battles cancer. It will help you understand things he or she may not know or may be uncomfortable discussing with you. It is also designed to inform you about ways to support him or her.

Cancer strikes across age levels, but it is certainly not the death sentence that it once was. Keeping on top of it with a proactive attitude is a good way to start. By learning all you can, you will help overcome your distress and better be able to use your energy fighting the disease.

Disclaimer

As with any book on a medical topic, if you believe you have cancer or if you have been diagnosed with cancer, obtain professional medical advice.

This book contains only general information on radiation therapy and chemotherapy. It is not the intention of the author or publisher to replace the advice of a healthcare professional or other healthcare provider. If you believe you have cancer or if you have been diagnosed with cancer, it is of utmost importance to obtain professional medical advice in order to receive not only a proper diagnosis but also effective treatment. At the time this book went to press, all of the information it contained was accurate. However, the national recommendations and guidelines that this book was based upon can change at any time. Please check with your health-care professional before using the information in this book.

'It is not the intention of the author or publisher to replace the advice of a healthcare professional or other healthcare provider.'

Chapter One
Treating Cancer

What is cancer?

The smallest living part of your body is called a cell. During a normal life cycle, each cell divides, carries out the things necessary for life and then dies. If you look at your skin, for example, you can see the dead skin cells that you clean away when you bathe. The renewing of cells keeps the body healthy.

'When your body is working correctly, the DNA tells cells to divide and make more cells when there is space around them.'

Each cell has a set of directions inside it called DNA. These directions tell the cell when to make new cells by dividing, what jobs they need to do in your body, and when to die. When your body is working correctly, the DNA tells cells to divide and make more cells when there is space around them. It tells them to stop dividing when they get crowded, and it may tell them to die if they are too closely packed together. It also tells old cells or cells that are not doing their job right to die.

Some things can cause the directions to get mixed-up, to lose parts or to have errors. Since your cells are constantly making more of themselves, this can happen naturally when they are copying the directions for a new cell. Or it can happen when something, such as too much direct sunlight, changes the directions. Sometimes people are born with mixed up directions. When the directions get muddled, the cell may keep dividing even when it is too cramped. It may not die even when it is not working right. When cells with jumbled directions build up, they form a mass called a tumor.

One type of tumor is called a benign tumor. These can be removed with surgery and usually do not come back. Most importantly, benign tumors do not spread to other parts of the body, and they are not life threatening.

Malignant tumors can be life threatening. These tumors grow and divide out of control. They stop resembling the cells they are supposed to be (i.e. skin cells, bone cells) and become undifferentiated or lose their particular characteristics. Once these cells stop looking like the cells around them, they can spread to other parts of your body. They can travel through your bloodstream or lymphatic system to other areas. Normally, these systems remove toxins from your body and fight disease, but the undifferentiated cells confuse them. When these pieces of the tumor metastasize or move to other parts of the body, they can begin to grow in that new area.

'Malignant tumors can be life threatening.'

The four types of malignant tumors.

Malignant tumors are classified based on the tissue or group of similar cells that they originally came from. There are four types of malignant tumors:

- Carcinomas: The tumor is formed from epithelial tissue or skin tissue that lines or covers organs or the body.

- Sarcomas: The tumor begins in connective tissue or the bone and cartilage that connects and supports the body.

- Lymphomas: Tumors that originate in the lymphatic system or the system that helps your body fight disease.

- Leukemia: When tumors begin in the blood.

What cancer cells do differently

Cancer cells have a set of directions that do not allow the cell to operate normally. These are some differences between normal cells and cancer cells:

'Cancer cells have a set of directions that do not allow the cell to operate normally.'

- Normal cells tell themselves to stop growing at a certain point. Cancer cells tell themselves to keep growing.

- Normal cells stop growing when the cells next to them tell them they are getting too big. Cancer cells keep growing even when neighboring cells tell them to stop.

- Groups of cancer cells make new blood vessels within them to bring the tumor nutrients and oxygen and to remove waste. This process is called angiogenesis.

- Normal cells kill themselves when they stop doing their job. Cancer cells do not kill themselves although they do not do the job they are supposed to do.

Where cancer begins

Because cancer cells are just a normal cells that have bad directions, cancer can begin anywhere in the body and move to anywhere in the body. However, cancer is classified by where it originally began and what type of cell it originally was. Survival rates are calculated based on this classification. The following are the standard kinds of cancer:

- Bladder cancer

- Bone and connective tissue cancers

- Colorectal cancer (cancer of the intestines)

- Brain tumors

- Breast cancer

- Cervical cancer (cancer of a woman's cervix)

- Hodgkin's lymphoma (cancer of the lymphatic system)

- Kidney cancer

- Laryngeal cancer (cancer of the larynx or voice box)

- Leukemia (cancer of the blood)

- Liver cancer

- Lung cancer

'...cancer can begin anywhere in the body and move to anywhere in the body.'

- Mesothelioma (tumor that began in the lining of body cavities)

- Myeloma (cancer of plasma cells in the blood)

- Non-Hodgkin lymphoma (cancer of the lymphatic system)

- Esophageal cancer (cancer of the throat)

- Oral cancer (cancer of the mouth)

- Ovarian cancer (cancer of a woman's ovary)

'Internal factors [that cause cancer] are things inside your body that you cannot change.'

- Pancreatic cancer (cancer of the pancreas)

- Prostate cancer (cancer of a man's prostate)

- Skin cancer

- Stomach cancer

- Testicular cancer (cancer of a man's testicle)

- Uterine cancer (cancer of the womb)

- Vaginal cancer (cancer of a woman's vagina)

- Vulval cancer (cancer of a woman's vulva)

What causes damage to DNA?

Both internal and external things can cause damage to the directions in your cell. Internal factors are things inside your body that you cannot change, and they include:

- Genetic factors: sometimes you are born with damaged DNA.

- Hormones: since hormones work directly with your DNA, they can cause damage to it.

- Age: as you get older, your cells have to divide more and more. As each new copy of the directions is made, your chances of developing cancer increase.

- Lowered immune system: your immune system fights cancer to some extent. If you have an illness that lowers or attacks your immune system, you have an increased chance of developing cancer.

'Try to quit smoking and to avoid secondhand smoke.'

- Prior cancer: Once you have had cancer, your chances of getting it again rise.

External factors are related to things outside your body that you can influence:

- Tobacco: try to quit smoking and to avoid secondhand smoke.

- Hormone supplements: if you need supplements, stay on them for the shortest period of time possible.

- Unhealthy diet and a sedentary lifestyle: obesity increases your chances of having cancer. Eat sensibly and get regular exercise to reduce your risk.

- Exposure to the sun's radiation: Sunlight affects DNA directly. Be sure to protect your skin when you are outside.

- Excessive drinking of alcohol: Try to limit your alcohol consumption to no more than one drink per day. If you are having difficulty limiting your drinking, speak to your health care provider for suggestions about it.

- Exposure to cancer causing chemicals: Some chemicals, such as pesticides, damage your DNA. Try to avoid using these chemicals and wear protective gear if you cannot avoid them.

'Many different procedures are used to make a complete diagnosis...'

- Infections: Some viruses and other infections can increase your chances of getting cancer. Keep your vaccinations up-to-date.

- Sexual and lifestyle behaviors: Some STDs can cause cancer. Also, certain recreational drugs can increase your chances for cancer. Talk to your healthcare professional about ways to reduce your risks.

How is cancer diagnosed?

Once a tumor is potentially detected through self-examination, screening, or a visit to your doctor, it is important for your doctor to make a complete cancer diagnosis. Many different procedures are used to make a complete diagnosis, and you may have to have one or more of these:

- Biopsy: A piece of the tumor is removed and a pathologist looks at the tissue under a microscope to determine if it looks malignant or benign.

- General X-ray: Although this technique has been around for a long time, it is highly effective in finding tumors.

- Blood tests: These not only monitor cancer, but also they give your healthcare professional an inside look at your overall health and the way your body is responding to treatment.

- CT scans: Computerized tomography (CT) scans use moving X-rays to create a three dimensional image.

- Mammogram: A specialized X-ray used for detecting breast cancer.

- MRI scan: a magnetic resonance imaging (MRI) scan uses a strong magnetic field to detect differences between soft tissues in your body from signals sent out by the water your body contains.

- Nuclear medicine: a small amount of radioactive material is injected into the body and travels to certain areas allowing the doctor to assess how those areas are functioning.

- PET scan: a positron emission tomography scan is used in combination with a CT scan to create better imaging. It uses a radioactive material, usually the sugar

'Be assured that your doctor is only asking you to undertake what is necessary for proper diagnosis and treatment.'

glucose, that is broken down by normal cells. It is able to detect cancer cells because they use glucose differently.

- Ultrasound: creates pictures of organs, muscles, fluid filled spaces, and bone surfaces using sound waves.

- Lab tests: the urine, stool, pus, etc. samples are analyzed to determine if the patient has infection or abnormal bleeding.

'There are many different treatments that doctors can use, and in some cases, you may have treatment options.'

Sometimes these tests need to be repeated either during treatment or to clear up conflicting information. Be assured that your doctor is only asking you to undertake what is necessary for proper diagnosis and treatment.

How do healthcare professionals treat cancer?

The way healthcare professionals treat cancer depends on many factors:

- The kind of cancer it is.

- How old you are.

- How healthy you are.

- Where the cancer is.

- You medical history.

- If the cancer is in more than one part of your body.

There are many different treatments that doctors can use, and in some cases, you may have treatment options. Your healthcare professionals may combine any of these treatments:

- Biological therapies: These use things that would naturally be found in your body, such as vaccines and genes, to fight cancer.

- Hormonal therapies: These therapies affect your hormones, which affect cell activity and growth. Changing the hormone levels in your body sometimes influences cancer cells.

- Surgery: This removes the cancer mass from the body. Frequently, chemotherapy, radiation, or both are used after surgery to destroy or contain cancer cells that may remain.

- Radiation: Uses high-energy rays to destroy cancer cells.

- Chemotherapy: Uses chemicals to destroy cancer cells.

- Stem cell and/or bone marrow transplants: Removes cancer and replaces it with stem cells.

- Supportive therapies: Supportive therapies are given with other cancer treatments to help reduce the symptoms and side effects the primary treatment may cause. An example would be a blood transfusion.

'Supportive therapies are given with other cancer treatments to help reduce the symptoms and side effects the primary treatment may cause.'

- Other rare therapies: These treatments may require that you travel because only a few hospitals have them available. They include hyperbaric oxygen therapy (HBOT), which uses extra oxygen to combat severe side effects of treatment, photodynamic therapy (PDT), which uses light to fight cancer, and radiofrequency ablation (RFA), which uses radio waves to fight cancer.

What is the difference between radiation therapy and chemotherapy?

'Radiation uses high-energy rays to destroy cancer cells. Chemotherapy uses medicines or chemicals to destroy cancer cells.'

Radiation therapy uses high-energy particles to penetrate tissues and cancer cells. These particles can be projected in a beam that is aimed directly at the cancer, or they can be released from implanted radioactive seeds. Radiation therapy targets the area where the cancer is or was. Radiation therapy must be done at the hospital or clinic.

Chemotherapy uses medicines or chemicals to fight cancer. Any drug or drug combination that slows, damages, or kills the cancer can be considered chemotherapy. Chemotherapy affects the entire body and works well at destroying cancer cells that may have moved away from the original tumor. Chemotherapy targets your entire body. Chemotherapy is done at the hospital, at the clinic, or at home.

Whether you get radiation therapy, chemotherapy, or both depends on the type of cancer you have, your treatment plan, where your cancer is, and how healthy you are in general. It is also important for your doctor to determine if your cancer remained in one place or if it moved to other parts of your body. Aside from surgery, radiation therapy and chemotherapy are the two most prescribed treatments for cancer.

What is a treatment plan?

The plan of action for fighting your cancer is called a treatment plan. Your doctors will first find all the information out about your cancer and your current state of health before developing a treatment plan. In addition to this, your treatment plan will be based upon other factors including your age, sex, family history, parts of the body affected by the cancer, lifestyle, other medical problems, and other medicines you are currently taking. During your course of treatment, your team of doctors may adjust this plan as they monitor your progress and determine your body's response to it.

'The plan of action for fighting your cancer is called a treatment plan.'

Making your treatment plan more effective

The first thing you can do to play an active part in your treatment and make it more effective is to create a treatment file folder with dividers and extra paper for recording symptoms, side effects, notes and questions. Write questions and side effects (including date and time) down as you have them and take them with you to the doctor. Write the answers to these questions right in your file.

Other things you need to keep in your file include:

- Notes from your appointments.

- A list of the names of all your consulting doctors along with what they specialize in and their contact information.

- A calendar for recording appointments.

- A list of all the medications you are on, the dosages, how frequently you take them and the number of treatments you have had.

- Record all important phone numbers (doctors, nurses, pharmacists, etc.) and write down to whom they belong.

- All your copies of lab work, test results, and any information your healthcare professionals give you.

- All the information about your treatments and information about side effects.

- If you find any information about community resources, helpful websites, classes, support groups, and other helpful resources, they can go in this file, too.

'Write questions and side effects (including date and time) down as you have them and take them with you to the doctor.'

A well organized and updated file will give you all the information you need at your fingertips without giving you the added stress of trying to memorize it.

In addition to creating a treatment file, you may also find it useful to create a blog that journals your feelings, the things you have learned and helpful resources you have found. Not only will this allow you to get your thoughts down and record them, but it will also help you to share the information with family and friends in an easy format. By saving a copy, you will create a record of your journey. If you prefer, you could keep a traditional journal instead.

When you visit your doctors, it is helpful to bring someone with you to help remember the information and to help you take notes. It is also a good idea to repeat the instructions that the doctor gives you back to him or her. This ensures that you have understood them correctly.

Questions for your doctor

Some good questions to ask your doctor when you are beginning treatment are:

- Is the goal of my treatment to get rid of the cancer, slow the spread of the cancer, relieve my symptoms or prevent the cancer from returning?

- Will I need other treatment?

- What are the names of the chemotherapy medications I will be using?

- What kind of radiation treatment will I need?

- How many treatments will I need? How frequent will they be? How long will each one last?

- What side effects may I experience? What can I do to prevent them?

'A well organized and updated file will give you all the information you need at your fingertips without giving you the added stress of trying to memorize it.'

- Will my treatments affect my sexual desire and/or fertility? Is this effect permanent or temporary?

- What tests will I need during the treatment?

- Will the treatment affect my other medical conditions? Will there be any interactions with the other medicines or herbs I take?

What are clinical trials?

'Even if you are invited to take part in a clinical trial, you are never obligated to do so.'

The key to discovering new, more effective treatments for cancer lies in testing new treatments on controlled groups. Studies on new types of treatments or new ways of using old treatments are run by universities, government organizations, and hospitals. The results of these studies are then published so the methods can continue to be tested and adjusted in order to create cancer treatments with maximum effectiveness. The goal is to have a successful treatment that creates fewer side effects or milder side effects and that is less disruptive to normal cell activity. In addition, researchers seek to find treatments that are more efficient at targeting and killing cancer cells or slowing their growth. Also, researchers want to find treatments that are more convenient for patients to have, require fewer appointments, or allow for a quicker recovery. Sometimes clinical studies simply show that the traditional treatment is the better one.

You may be invited to a clinical trial, or your doctor may recommend one for you. If you are interested in learning about clinical trials, there are several agencies that are involved in clinical trials for people with cancer:

- National Cancer Institute (NCI)

- American Cancer Society (ACS)

Even if you are invited to take part in a clinical trial, you are never obligated to do so. And before you participate, all the benefits and risks will be explained to you, as well as possible side effects you may experience from the treatment. You will be able to ask questions about the trial. Just keep in mind that the treatments anyone undergoes now were once past clinical trials. Any clinical trials you take part in will improve the treatment of future generations.

'When you visit your doctors, it is helpful to bring someone with you to help remember the information and to help you take notes.'

Summing Up

- Cancer is a malignant tumor that grows and divides abnormally without dying because its DNA has an error in it.

- Cancer is classified based on where it first appears and the type of tissue in which it first appears.

- Internal factors that you cannot control and external factors that you can control both cause damage to your DNA that can lead to cancer.

- Cancer is diagnosed through a series of tests that your doctor will set up for you. These same tests will be used throughout your treatment to monitor your response.

Sometimes these tests need to be repeated for better results.

- Healthcare professionals will treat your cancer based on the type of cancer you have and your unique and individual situation.

- Radiation therapy uses a high-energy beam to treat the area where the cancer is or was. Chemotherapy uses medicines to treat your entire body for cancer.

'Create an organized file that contains all the information about your doctors and treatment.'

- Your treatment plan is designed by your doctor for your unique case. Keeping a treatment file will help you organize your life and increase the effectiveness of your treatment.

- Create an organized file that contains all the information about your doctors and treatment.

- You may be referred to or invited to a clinical trial. These trials are important ways of discovering better treatments.

Chapter Two
Radiation Therapy

How does radiation therapy work?

Radiation therapy works by depositing high levels of energy in the tissue and cells that make up the tissue as it passes through them. This either kills the cancer cells or breaks the DNA inside them so they stop growing, dividing, and spreading to other areas of the body. Although the radiation can also break the DNA in nearby cells that are normal, they generally are able to repair themselves because they are working like they should. Since the DNA is already damaged in cancer cells, they are not able to repair the damage done by the radiation.

The total amount of radiation you need is divided into fractions or parts. Each treatment you have gives you one of these fractions of radiation. Sometimes the treatments themselves are called fractions. Since radiation accumulates in your system with exposure, this allows doctors to reduce the side effects caused by high levels of radiation while providing you with enough radiation to damage or kill the cancer cells.

'[It] either kills the cancer cells or breaks the DNA inside them so they stop growing, dividing and spreading to other areas of the body.'

Why are there different kinds of radiation therapy?

Since every case in unique, radiation therapy needs to be tailored to the type of tumor, the overall health of the patient, and the location of the cancer. For example, radioisotope therapy works by attaching a radioactive particle to a drug that concentrates the radioactivity in the affected organ, such as your thyroid. If your cancer is in another part of your body, this method will not work. One the other hand, brachytherapy or internal therapy works well if a beam of radiation would need to penetrate several layers of tissue to reach the affected area.

All types of radiation therapy are used for destroying cancer, slowing its growth, and relieving symptoms of cancer. However, your doctors will be able to determine which kind of radiation therapy or what combination of radiation therapy techniques will work best for you. In general, radiation therapy techniques are classified as external and internal depending on the source of the radiation.

'External radiation therapy is one of the most common forms of radiation therapy.'

What is external radiation therapy?

External radiation therapy is one of the most common forms of radiation therapy. The equipment needed for this kind of therapy is large because it sends out high-intensity radiation, usually in the form of X-rays. However, these X-rays are thousands of times stronger than what you would experience with a general X-ray. Gamma rays, protons, and ions are other types of radiation that may be used. You will be placed in a certain position, and the machine will move around you to send the radiation directly where it is needed. The machine will target the area from several angles to make sure it has gotten everything. Treatment itself is not painful, but side effects may develop later.

Usually you receive external radiation therapy over several weeks. You generally go in each day during the week and have weekends off. However, you can go in three days a week, every day including weekends, or even more than once a day. Each treatment takes only a few minutes, but it can take up to 15 minutes to get ready and get in the proper position. The machine may or may not touch you during the therapy. After your normal scheduled sessions are finished, you may have some brief treatments just to the area where the tumor was. External radiation does not make you radioactive, so it is safe to be around friends and family afterward.

There will be several doctors involved in your radiation therapy treatment. A clinical oncologist (cancer specialist) who specializes in radiation therapy, a medical physicist, and a therapeutic radiologist will devote their skills to your case.

'There will be several doctors involved in your radiation therapy treatment.'

There are many types of external radiation you could undergo:

- Image-guided radiation therapy (IGRT) uses imaging techniques in addition to the radiation therapy in order to confirm the tumor is being properly targeted.

- Conformal or intensity-modulated radiation therapy (IMRT) uses radiation therapy beams to give a very precise dose of radiation. These beams are shaped to conform precisely to the shape of the tumor, which reduces side effects.

- Volumetric modulated arc therapy (VMAT) is a newer method of external radiation therapy. Sometimes this is also called RapidArc® radiation therapy depending on the manufacturer of the equipment being used. This type of radiation therapy uses three-dimensional imaging techniques to help pinpoint the area being radiated. The ability to control the radiation delivery is highly accurate with this method.

- Stereotactic radiation therapy uses many beams of radiation to target the tumor from several angles. Because a lower dose beam is used, the surrounding tissues get less radiation (in theory) than the tumor. CyberKnife® and Gamma Knife® are the names given to these machines by two different manufacturers.

'Total body irradiation (TBI) is only used for people receiving stem cell transplants.'

- Total body irradiation (TBI) is only used for people receiving stem cell transplants. It can be done in one large dose or up to eight smaller doses. It is frequently used in combination with chemotherapy. Once the treatment is finished, stem cells that will become blood cells and platelets are given to the patient. These may come from the patient or from a donor.

- Intra-operative radiation or radiosurgery combines surgery to remove the tumor with radiation delivered during the surgery to allow doctors to pinpoint small, well-defined tumors.

- Proton beam therapy (PBT) is for rare cancers, especially those affecting children. Energized protons (the center of an atom) are shot at the tumor. With this therapy, damage to the surrounding, healthy cells is minimal. Insurance companies may not cover this new treatment, or they may only cover it for certain cancer diagnosis.

What is brachytherapy?

Brachytherapy is a type of internal radiation therapy. A solid source of radiation is implanted in your body directly in or near the tumor. The radiation sources for this kind of radiation therapy are usually iodine-131, strontium-89, caesium-131 or technetium-99. Inserting the radiation can be done at the same time a tumor is removed or it can be performed as a separate procedure. Because the process involves a minor surgery, you may need some sort of anesthetic during the implantation process. The process may or may not require you to stay in the hospital.

'Brachy-therapy is a type of internal radiation therapy.'

The rods, pellets, or seeds of radioactive materials are placed and then removed a few minutes, a few days, a few months later. In some cases they may not be removed. With internal radiation, you can emit radiation from your body that will affect others. Talk with your doctor to find out if you will need to avoid anyone, such as pregnant women, during your treatment or if there are certain restrictions on your movements.

There are two types of brachytherapy you could undergo:

- Low dose rate brachytherapy (also called implant brachytherapy, seed implant brachytherapy, or pinhole surgery) is when your clinical oncologist implants between 80 and 120 small, radioactive seeds into the tumor or near it. Since the radiation does not travel far in the body, it can be left in until the radiation fades from the seeds.

- High dose rate brachytherapy is usually done in combination with a form of external radiation therapy. For this treatment, thin tubes containing radioactive material are inserted into the tumor area. The tubes are left in for as long as they need to be to achieve the correct dose. When the doctor removes the tubes, there is no radiation left in your body. The dose is higher than you receive with low dose rate brachytherapy, but the tubes are left in for a much shorter period of time.

'Radio-isotope therapy uses a source that is delivered less invasively through a drink or capsules, or by injection into a vein.'

What is radioisotope therapy (RIT)?

Radioisotope therapy is another internal radiation therapy. However, instead of implanting a solid radiation source, radioisotope therapy uses a source that is delivered less invasively through a drink or capsules or by injection into a vein. The radiation source for this form of radiation therapy is usually iodine, but it may also be strontium depending on your cancer. You will need to stay in the hospital for this procedure until radiation levels inside your body fall to safe levels.

Like other forms of internal radiation therapy, you can emit radiation for a while after treatment. You will be kept in the hospital for up to seven days as this radiation dissipates, but once you leave, you may still need to avoid certain people, such as children for some time. Talk with your doctor or hospital staff so you can understand the precautions you will need to take and how long you will need to take them.

What will I need to do to prepare before having radiation therapy?

You will need to attend treatment-planning sessions. Ask your radiologist how long these will last because they can take up to an hour. During this time, the doctor or radiologist will help position you so you can receive the best treatment. You will need to resume this same position for each treatment, but the staff will help you with it. In addition, the doctor or radiologist will make marks on your body in permanent ink or with a more permanent tattoo. Please try not to wash off or remove these marks until you are told you may, or you will need another treatment planning session to re-mark them.

If you need radiation therapy to your head or neck, you will need to have a special mask made to keep your head still during treatment. You should shave facial hair and trim or cut long hair for this process. Keep your hair cut during treatment to ensure the mask continues to fit in the same way. Plan to spend at least 30 minutes in the mold department to have a mask made. You may need a second visit to make adjustments. This mask will be made from Perspex or mesh plastic. It will allow the Radiologists to make marks directly on it in order to pinpoint treatment areas. You will only need to wear the mask during the planning session(s) and the treatments. However, the mask will be secured to

'You will need to attend treatment-planning sessions before you have radiation therapy.'

the table so that you do not move during those times. Remember the treatments will only take a few minutes, and the staff will be nearby should you have any questions.

What should I expect when I go for radiation therapy treatment?

Different things will happen based on the type of radiation therapy you are having. However, you will do the same things each time.

External radiation.

You will need to put on a hospital gown on at the beginning of each treatment session. You will go to a special radiation therapy room where you can lie on a couch in the same position you were shown during the planning sessions. The radiation machine will be above you. If you are having treatment to your head or neck, you will put on your mask and be secured to the table. The therapist will adjust your position as needed and position the machine properly. You may or may not have lead shields placed on your body to protect unaffected body parts from the radiation.

'You will do the same things each time.'

As soon as you and the machine are properly positioned, the therapist will leave you and go to a separate control room. This room protects them from repeated radiation exposure. They will still be able to see you and hear you, so if you need to talk with them you can. Over the course of a few minutes, the therapist will administer the radiation. Sometimes, you, the machine or both will need to be repositioned so the radiation can pass through your body at a different angle.

Each time you have a treatment, you will follow these steps again: You will change into the gown; you and the machine will be positioned; the radiation will be administered while the therapist is in the control room.

Brachytherapy.

Like external radiation, you may need planning sessions so the doctor can map out where the radiation will be placed. However, these will consist of scans and imaging appointments. When you go in for treatment, you will be placed under general anesthesia or you will receive a spinal (epidural). The material will then be inserted with a surgical procedure.

In some cases, you will be allowed to go home. In others, you will need to stay in the hospital until the material is removed. You may also need a catheter (a tube inserted into your bladder to allow your urine to drain without using the restroom), and you may need to lie in bed during the treatment to prevent the material from dislodging. For treatments that involve the mouth, you will only be able to eat liquid foods and may be fed through a tube. You may also have limited access to visitors in order to reduce their exposure to the radiation.

'Once your treatment is complete, the radioactive material will be removed and the applicators will be removed.'

Once your treatment is complete, the radioactive material will be removed, and any applicators will be removed. Any catheters or feeding tubes will also be removed. You will receive painkillers to help with any pain or discomfort you may have. Once the radioactive material is removed, you will no longer emit radiation, so you will be able to return home the same day or the day afterward.

Radioisotope therapy.

When you receive radioisotopes as a part of internal radiation therapy, you will need to stay in the hospital. Plan to stay a week, but you may get to return home earlier if you drink plenty of fluids. Fluids will help flush the radioactivity out of your body through your urine and sweat.

In some cases, you may need to avoid young children and pregnant women for a time after your treatment. You may also have blood or urine that is slightly radioactive for few days. Please be sure to inquire about any precautions you should take when you leave the hospital, and then follow them.

"When you receive radio-isotopes as a part of internal radiation therapy... plan to stay [in the hospital] a week.'

What is new in this field?

In addition to working with the latest radiation therapy machines to discover how to use them more effectively, there are many trials underway to see how to best combine internal and external radiation therapy methods, what the best dosages are for radiation therapy, and how to best combine radiation therapy with other cancer treatments.

Hyperfractionated radiation therapy focuses on giving your radiation therapy treatments over the course of 12 days instead of several weeks. This is a new therapy being tested that would require you to stay in the hospital because you would receive more than one treatment per day. However, it drastically would shorten the length of time that you were receiving treatments.

Hypofractionated radiation therapy is when doctors use higher dosages of radiation per fraction but a lower overall dose by giving fewer treatments.

Other new methods that are currently being researched are using antibodies to deliver radioactive materials directly to cancer cells, using oxygen therapy (HBO) to reduce bowel problems after pelvic radiation therapy treatments, and using steroid cream to reduce the skin side effects.

Summing Up

- Radiation therapy works by killing cancer cells or breaking the DNA in cancer cells so that they no longer divide, grow, or spread.

- There are different types of radiation therapy so that different cancers and different cancer patients can be treated.

- External radiation is generated by a large machine and focused on the tumor. There are several methods for delivering this radiation: image-guided radiation therapy (IGRT), conformal or intensity-modulated radiation therapy (IMRT), volumetric modulated arc therapy (VMAT), stereotactic radiation therapy, total body irradiation (TBI), intra-operative radiation or radiosurgery, and proton beam therapy (PBT).

- Brachytherapy is when a solid, radioactive material is surgically inserted into the tumor

'There are different types of radiation therapy so that different cancers and different cancer patients can be treated.'

or near it. There are two general forms of brachytherapy: low dose rate and high dose rate.

- Radioisotope therapy delivers radioactive material usually in liquid form either orally or by injection. This material then accumulates in the affected organ.

- You will need a treatment planning session with your doctor. For external radiation, you may need to have a mask made if the radiation therapy is to be delivered to your head or neck. This will be done prior to your first treatment.

'There are many new methods of using radiation therapy that are currently being researched.'

- The treatment sessions will be similar to each other and will consist of you going to the hospital or clinic to receive your treatments and remaining there until the radiation is no longer in your body. You may need additional support with catheters, feeding tubes, etc. if you are having brachytherapy.

- There are many new methods of using radiation therapy that are currently being researched. In addition, some research is being directed at controlling or diminishing the side effects from radiation therapy treatments.

Chapter Three
Chemotherapy

How does chemotherapy work?

Chemotherapy uses chemicals that are cytotoxic medicines or medicines that are poisonous to dividing cells. Most normal cells do not divide to make new cells as frequently as cancer cells do. In fact, cancer cells are generally always dividing, and normal cells are not. Since chemotherapy works by damaging or interfering with cells that are dividing it is able to target cancer cells throughout the body.

There are many different cytotoxic medicines. However, they act on dividing cells in different ways and at different points during the division. They can kill cells that are dividing or at least stop them from continuing to divide and make more bad copies of themselves.

In order for chemotherapy to work, it must be able to enter the bloodstream and travel throughout the body. Since the chemotherapy drugs are able to reach any area of your body through the bloodstream, using them is considered a systemic approach to fighting cancer.

Although all chemotherapy medicines attack dividing cells, they each perform their job in different ways. The type of cancer you have and the stage of your cancer will help your doctor

'Since the chemo-therapy drugs are able to reach any area of your body through the blood-stream, using them is considered a systemic approach to fighting cancer.'

determine the type of chemotherapy medicine or the combination of chemotherapy medicines that will work best for you.

Although most normal cells, such as muscle cells, brain cells, and bone cells, do not divide frequently, a few normal cells do divide rapidly. The cells in your bone marrow constantly produce new blood cells. The cells of your hair constantly add length to it. Also, your skin cells are continuously making more cells. Because these cells are always replacing themselves, they are affected by chemotherapy drugs. This is why there are common chemotherapy side effects, such as you hair falling out.

'Because some cells are always replacing themselves, they are affected by chemo-therapy drugs.'

The benefit that normal dividing cells have over cancer cells is that normal cells can repair themselves quickly or replace cells that have been damaged badly. Cancer cells are not good at doing that. For this reason, your doctor may have you use a chemotherapy medicine, and then allow your normal cells a rest to repair themselves fully. Once they have had time to do that, you may begin to take chemotherapy again. The key is to ensure that the break is not too long. You do not want the cancer cells to have enough time to repair themselves.

Usually the treatments can last up to a week and the break can last up to four weeks. This cyclic treatment means that you will get your dose over a period of time and allow time for your normal cells to repair themselves before the next dose. One treatment period (a dose) of chemotherapy and one period of rest is called a cycle. All the cycles during your treatment collectively are referred to as a course of treatment and may last six months or so. It is important to follow your treatment plan and take your chemotherapy when your doctor has prescribed it; however, your doctor may change the treatment schedule from what was initially discussed based on how your body responds to it.

How do I get chemotherapy?

Although chemotherapy is generally given in a hospital or clinic, it can also be taken at home. There are four main ways chemotherapy can be given to you during your course of treatment. They are described below:

- *Injection into a vein (sometimes called an intravenous injection)*: This can be performed using a syringe and needle. It can also be done over several hours, several days or even several weeks by inserting a thin plastic tube into a vein in your arm and allowing a pump to maintain a steady rate of drip from a bag of diluted medicine. Sometimes the plastic tube is inserted into your chest or in a deeper vein and it is allowed to stay there throughout your treatment course. This method is becoming very popular since it only requires the tube to be inserted once. It also allows blood samples to be taken from the same tube. With this method, it is important to take special care of the line so that it will not become blocked or infected. The nurse will teach you or your caregiver how to clean it every week and provide you with a waterproof cover for when you take

'Although chemo-therapy is generally given in a hospital or clinic, it can also be taken at home.'

baths or showers. If you or your caregiver is unable to take care of the line, a nurse can be assigned to do it. You should also take care to keep scissors away from the line so it does not get cut. You will need to keep valves and clamps closed and caps in place when it is not in use. If you notice pain, redness, or swelling around the line, a discolored fluid leaking from or around it, or if you run a fever, contact your doctor right away. There are three methods that require care and should be watched for infection. These are called implantable ports, central lines, or PICC (peripherally inserted central catheters) lines. If one of these is placed in the arm, take care that you do not lift anything over 14 pounds with that arm and that your blood pressure is not taken from that arm.

'If you notice pain, redness or swelling around the line, a discolored fluid leaking from or around it, or if you run a fever, contact your doctor straight away.'

- Some chemotherapy medicines are given to you in the form of liquids or tablets that are made to be taken by mouth and absorbed into the blood stream through the stomach.

- If the chemotherapy needs to reach your brain or spinal cord, you may need a lumbar puncture. This is a small needle inserted into your lower back in the space next to the spinal cord. The reason some people need this method is because there is a filtering system that keeps most medicines in your blood from entering your brain and spinal cord.

- Sometimes, the medicine needs to be injected directly into a muscle, into your chest cavity, or into the tumor itself.

- Certain cytotoxic medicines are given as a cream that is rubbed into the skin.

What are alkylating agents?

Alkylating agents are chemotherapy drugs that work by targeting the DNA of cancer cells and preventing the cells from reproducing and growing. They do this by removing an active hydrogen atom from the DNA and placing an inactive molecule in its place. When this happens the DNA cannot separate into two copies of directions when the cell tries to divide. Instead the DNA is broken into pieces. The first alkylating agent used as chemotherapy was nitrogen mustard (from mustard gas). Cyclophosphamide, dacarbazine, and chlorambucil are some of the alkylating agents that are used today.

'Alkylating agents are chemotherapy drugs that work by targeting the DNA of cancer cells and preventing the cells from reproducing and growing.'

What are anthracyclines?

These chemotherapy drugs were first developed from antibiotics. They work by fitting between the strands of DNA and locking them together. When the DNA strands are wedged together like this, they cannot separate into the two sets of directions needed to make more cancer cells. Epirubicin and doxorubicin are the two most common drugs in this class, but bleomycin and mitomycin are also in this class of chemotherapy treatments.

What are anti-metabolites?

These were the second group of chemotherapy drugs to be developed. These drugs act by preventing DNA from making another copy of itself. When the copy of DNA directions is being made, they get added into it and make the list of directions end. This means the directions are shortened to the point of being useless. If DNA cannot copy itself, it cannot make more cancer cells. Methotrexate and fluorouracil are the oldest of this kind of drug, and they are still being used today. However, today fluorouricil is given with a vitamin (leucovorin) to increase the effectiveness of the drug. Modern drugs in this class are capecitabine (Xeloda®), fludarabine (Fludara®), gemcitabine (Gemzar®) and pemetrexed.

'...Today fluorouricil is given with a vitamin (leucovorin) to increase the effective-ness of the drug.'

What are topoisomerase inhibitors?

Topoisomerases are enzymes that help speed up the process when DNA is making more copies of itself. The topoisomerase inhibitors clamp onto the topoisomerases and prevent them from working. Because it would take a very long time for DNA to make copies without enzymes, topisomerase inhibitors stop new DNA from being made and halts cell division. Drugs from this class of chemotherapy include etoposide, topetecan (Hycamtin®) and irinotecan (Campto®).

What are plant alkaloids or spindle poisons?

Each cell has a structure of tubulin inside it that separates the parts of the cell when the cell divides. Spindle poisons destroy this structure so when the cell goes to divide it cannot pull itself apart. All spindle poisons are plant alkaloids. They come from natural compounds. Some of these plant compounds have been derived from the periwinkle plant (Vinca rosea). These include vinorelbine (Navelbine®), vincristine (Oncovin®) and vinblastine (Velbe®). Others come from the Pacific yew and include docetaxol (Taxotere®), and paclitaxel (Taxol®).

What are platinum compounds?

Platinum compounds were first discovered to cause cell death in experiments on bacteria in the late 1960s. These work similar to alkylating compounds by linking DNA strands to each other and preventing the DNA from separating to make a copy of itself. Examples of platinum compounds that are used commonly today are oxaliplatin (Eloxatin®), cisplatin and carboplatin (Paraplatin®).

What is combination therapy?

Combination therapy is when several chemotherapy drugs are given for treatment. Frequently drugs that affect different areas of cell division are given together to make the chemotherapy more effective. Many combinations have been developed and many more are being developed. Usually, they are referred to by the acronyms of the drugs that are being given. You can always ask your doctor about your specific combination therapy drugs; however, these are some of the more common regimens:

'Combination therapy is when more than one chemo-therapy drug is given for treatment.'

- CMF: cyclophosphamide, methotrexate, and fluorouracil.

- Epi-CMF: four courses of epirubicin alone and then four courses of CMF.

- FEC: fluorouracil, epirubicin, and cuclophosphamide.

- AC: Adriamycin (brand name for doxorubicin) and cyclophosphamide.

- MIC: itomycin, isfosfamide, and cisplatin

- BEP: bleomycin, etoposide, and cisplatin.

- ABVD: Adriamycin (doxorubicin), bleomycin, vinblastine, and dacarbazine.

- CHOP: cyclophosphamide, doxorubicin, oncovin (vincristine), and prednisolone (a steroid).

'Feel free to ask your healthcare professional if you have any questions. Never think that he or she is too busy to answer them.'

What will I need to do to prepare for chemotherapy?

Like radiation therapy, chemotherapy requires a team working to help you. You will have an oncologist and chemotherapy nurse. Feel free to ask these healthcare professionals if you have any questions. Never think that they are too busy to answer them. It is important that all your questions are answered before you begin treatment.

In addition to normal diagnostic tests, you will need special tests before beginning chemotherapy treatment. You will probably undergo a series of tests to see how your body is doing and how healthy you are. Tests that check your liver, kidneys, lungs, hearing, and heart may all be performed. These tests may be repeated during treatment to monitor how these organs are doing and ensure they are continuing to work well. You may also need to be tested for certain diseases such as hepatitis and HIV because these diseases can interfere with treatment or cause you to need an alternative treatment.

It is best to have a dental check-up before you begin your chemotherapy. If you need dental work during your treatment, you increase your chance of getting an infection from it.

Make sure your doctor is aware of all the vitamins, drugs, and supplements that you are taking before you begin your chemotherapy. Some of these can interfere with the chemotherapy drugs and make it less effective. Others may have a combining effect and make the drugs stronger than what your body needs or can handle.

'It is best to have a dental check-up before you begin your chemo-therapy.'

If you would like to have children after treatment, talk with your healthcare provider. Some chemotherapy drugs cause temporary or permanent infertility. You may need to store eggs or sperm before treatment if you want to have children afterward.

If you are on a course of treatment that will cause hair loss, you may want to invest in a wig before your hair is gone. There are a variety of wigs available that can match both your style and color of hair so there will be little difference in your appearance. Keep in mind that after a course of treatment, your natural hair may change in texture (curlier or straighter) and color, but these changes are usually slight.

Find someone to help you around the house on the days of your treatments and the days following your treatments. If you do not have close family or friends or if you are a caregiver for another person, you can ask the hospital social worker about finding help.

'Find someone to help you around the house on the days of your treatments and the days following your treatments.'

Speak with your employer or teachers if you are working or engaged in an education program. Make sure you can plan time off around your treatments.

If you have children, arrange not only for someone to help care for them during your chemotherapy, but also find an emergency person you can contact in case something happens and you need extra help on short notice. Again talk with a hospital social worker if you need help finding additional support.

What will happen at my chemotherapy treatment?

Usually, you will go to the hospital and only as an outpatient, but your length of stay will be determined by the type and number of tests you need, the assessment of your situation, what chemotherapy treatments you need and what needs to be done to prepare you for those treatments.

If you are told that you will only be a day patient, expect to spend 4 – 6 hours or longer in the treatment. Bring someone with you to pass the time, a book, or even something like knitting to keep you occupied.

When you arrive, you will begin with your tests and assessments. Some of these will include a blood test to check your blood count. There may be other tests to ensure you are well enough to have treatment. You will either see your doctor or nurse the day before your treatment or before your treatment begins on the day of your chemotherapy. Bring any questions you may have for them about the treatment plan with you. You will also have your chemotherapy prescription checked.

'Bring someone with you to pass the time, a book or even something like knitting to keep you occupied.'

The chemotherapy will be prepared by the hospital's pharmacy. This will take place sometime after your tests and assessment. If you had these assessments the day before, your prescription may have been prepared in advance.

Once you have been checked and had any questions answered, your treatment will be given to you. You may receive chemotherapy drugs to take home. Be sure to follow the instructions your healthcare providers give you. You will also set up your next appointment before leaving.

In the beginning of your chemotherapy treatment, you may need to stay in the hospital overnight. Also, you may need to stay if you are receiving several drugs or infusions. These situations may require a stay of up to 48–hours. If you need a longer admission, your healthcare professionals will explain the reason you need it to you.

If you are receiving your chemotherapy at home through a continuous infusion, you will still need to visit the hospital every few weeks for a regular check-up to ensure everything is going well. If you have any difficulties or questions, write them down and bring them to these check-ups.

Why did my doctor change my treatment plan?

'While you are undergoing chemo-therapy, your doctor will monitor your body for significant changes... with periodic blood tests.'

While you are undergoing chemotherapy, your doctor will monitor your body for significant changes in the function of your organs with periodic blood tests. If your doctor notices a problem, he or she will either delay your chemotherapy for a little while, lower the dose of chemotherapy you are receiving, or change the chemotherapy drug(s) you are getting.

Another common reason for delaying your treatment is that your white blood cells are lower than normal. This is a common side effect of chemotherapy, since blood cells are among the types of cells that must be constantly dividing to make more of themselves. They are affected more severely by chemotherapy drugs. Once your doctor sees that your blood cells have recovered, you will continue treatment.

Sometimes, your doctor may order tests to see if the cancer is responding to the chemotherapy treatments. If the results of these tests show that the cancer has not been responding as expected, your doctor may change your treatment plan so it will be more effective with a different chemotherapy drug.

During your chemotherapy treatment, a special occasion may arise that would be difficult to attend because of where it falls in your treatment cycle. If this is the case, you can speak with your doctor. Although it is not always possible, sometimes treatments can be delayed so you can participate.

What is new in this field?

New drugs and new combinations of drugs are being introduced regularly to help reduce side effects and improve their effectiveness. In addition, new methods of giving chemotherapy are also being researched. If you are interesting in testing new chemotherapy drugs or methods of using chemotherapy, ask your doctor if you would be a candidate for any clinical trials.

Summing Up

- Chemotherapy works by attacking and killing cells that are dividing. Since cancer cells divide frequently and most of the other cells in your body do not, cancer cells are targeted through this treatment.

- You can receive chemotherapy by injection into a vein, orally, through a lumbar injection, injected directly into a muscle, injected into your chest cavity, injected into the tumor itself or as a cream.

- Alkylating agents are chemotherapy drugs that stop DNA from making copies of itself.

New drugs and new combinations of drugs are being introduced regularly to help reduce side effects and improve their effectiveness.

- Anthracyclines are chemotherapy drugs that lock strands of DNA together and prevent it from dividing.

- Anti-metabolites are chemotherapy drugs that stop DNA from making a copy of itself.

- Topoisomerase inhibitors prevent topoisomerases from helping to copy DNA quickly. This stops the cells from dividing.

- Spindle poisons or plant alkaloids break the structure within the cell so that the DNA and cell material cannot divide into two new cells.

'Anthra-cyclines are chemo-therapy drugs that lock strands of DNA together and prevent it from dividing.'

- Platinum compounds bind DNA together so that it cannot separate to make a copy of itself.

- Combination therapy is when several different chemotherapy drugs are used as a part of the chemotherapy treatment.

- Prepare for your chemotherapy treatment by undergoing any recommended tests, clearing time in your schedule to rest, and informing your doctor of other drugs, vitamins, and supplements you may be taking.

- Your doctor may change or delay your treatment plan to allow your body to recuperate or to better attack the cancer.

- New drugs, combinations of drugs and methods for administering drugs are being researched.

Chapter Four
Are There Side Effects?

What side effects can I expect after radiation therapy?

Because each person is unique different people may undergo different side effects even if they have the same type of radiation therapy. Below are some general side effects of radiation therapy:

- Fatigue: In general, the most common side effect of radiation therapy is being tired. You may not feel tired until after you have completed all your treatments.

- Localized hair loss: Unlike chemotherapy, radiation therapy may only create hair loss in the area of treatment.

- Skin burns, blisters, pain, peeling, or irritation: you may experience symptoms similar to sunburn at the site of radiation treatment.

- Lowered blood counts: high levels of radiation may reduce the number blood cells you have and increase your chances of infection or anemia.

- Joint stiffness or muscle aches: you may experience pain or stiffness in your joints or

'Because each person is unique different people may undergo different side effects even if they have the same type of radiation therapy.'

muscles up to two years after your treatment has concluded.

- Sexual and reproductive issues: radiation can temporarily or permanently damage fertility. In addition, women or men having radiation therapy on their sexual organs may find sex to be painful due to scarring. Men may become impotent.

Beyond these general side effects, there are other side effects that you could experience depending on the area of your body that is receiving the radiation.

'If the headache is severe, if you notice that your vision is changing, or if you are violently vomiting, you should contact your doctor right away.'

Head

- Headache. Because the brain retains water after radiation treatment, it swells just enough to create pressure. There is medication to deal with this, but if the headache is severe or you notice that your vision is changing or you are violently vomiting, you should contact your doctor right away.

- Sleepiness, confusion, or disorientation 1–3 hours after treatment. This occurs usually after the first treatment. If you take a nap, the symptoms usually go away when you wake up.

- Hair loss that can become permanent if the dose of radiation you need is high, the duration of treatment is long, or the number of treatments is high.

- Thickened saliva and loss of taste or altered ability to taste. These symptoms tend to get worse over the course of treatment. Use saliva replacements, analgesic gels for mouth sores, and hard candies to combat symptoms. Drink plenty of fluids and if your appetite fades, drink nutritional shakes.

Chest

- Swelling in the esophagus. This may cause discomfort when eating as food passes the swollen area or it may cause indigestion. Eat only lukewarm food, chew well, and avoid spicy foods and alcohol to help reduce symptoms.

- Excessive coughing and mucus. Talk with your doctor about non-prescription drugs you can take to alleviate these symptoms. Consider a vaporizer or sitting in the bathroom with the steam from the shower.

'Some people find mint, lemon, or ginger candies or teas help alleviate nausea.'

Upper abdomen (above the navel)

- Nausea. In addition to medicine your doctor may prescribe, some people find mint, lemon, or ginger candies or teas alleviate problems.

- Indigestion. This can be controlled by what you eat, and the doctor can give you medication for it.

- Loss of appetite. Always treat abdomen problems to prevent losing your appetite. If you do lose your appetite, there are nutritional shakes that you should drink to keep up your strength.

Lower abdomen (below the navel)

- Diarrhea. No matter how radiation is angled, it will pass through the intestines. As a result, it only takes a couple of weeks before this symptom may occur. Controlling diarrhea is important for maintaining your overall health. Speak with your healthcare provider for medications you can take to resolve this issue. Some people also find eating a banana or two each day is helpful.

- Rectum (rectum) irritation. Spasms and anus irritation can be treated with topical creams or suppositories. Talk with your doctor if you are experiencing these symptoms.

- Bladder spasms. If you feel like you constantly have to urinate and little comes out when you do, you may have a bladder spasm. Again, your doctor can provide medication to alleviate your symptoms.

'Controlling diarrhea is important for maintaining your overall health.'

What side effects can I expect from chemotherapy?

Just as each person may experience different side effects from radiation, they may also experience different side effect from chemotherapy. Each chemotherapy drug has different side effects associated with it. Talk with your healthcare provider to find out more information about the side effects of the drugs you are taking. However, in general, there are some overall chemotherapy side effects that occur with most of the drugs:

- Fatigue: Tiredness is common with chemotherapy as well as radiation. It is possible that there is a medical reason behind your weariness if you are taking chemotherapy. Talk to your doctor to be sure that your fatigue is not caused by hormonal imbalances, low levels of nutrients, or anemia. Your healthcare provider should be able to help resolve your tiredness.

- Hair loss: Hair loss is more common with chemotherapy than it is with radiation therapy. It can extend to your eyebrows, eyelashes, and other body hair. However, chemotherapy related hair loss is usually temporary and some women even find their hair growing back before treatment is complete.

- Lowered blood counts: Chemotherapy not only affects your entire system, it also attacks dividing cells, such as blood cells. For this reason, it is not only common for blood counts to be low, but doctors monitor chemotherapy patients for low blood counts. Always get blood tests done when your doctor recommends you have them. Make sure your doctor is aware of all supplements, vitamins, and medications (even ones you purchased without a prescription) that you are taking. This will help prevent internal bleeding which can contribute to low blood counts.

- Nausea and vomiting: With the anti-sickness drugs (anti-emetics) available

'Chemo-therapy related hair loss is usually temporary and some women even find their hair growing back before treatment is complete.'

today, this no longer needs to be an issue. Untreated, nausea can begin a few hours after chemotherapy is given, last for 2–4 days, and it can be severe enough to cause a person to vomit. Treated, you may feel a bit nauseous and queasy for a day or so, but that is all.

- Sore mouth. This occurs a few days after chemotherapy has been given and can last a week. Some people have minor discomfort, others develop painful mouth ulcers. If you have this symptom, you can lose your sense of taste or your sense of taste can be altered. Ask the nurse if you can suck or chew on ice 30 minutes before your chemotherapy, during it, and 30 minutes after it. This helps some people. Change your diet so you avoid foods that are acidic, salty, and spicy or foods that contain spirits such as gin. Change your toothpaste to one for sensitive mouths. Use a pain dulling mouthwash, gel, paste, or spray. Since your white blood cell count may also be low, it is possible to develop a yeast infection called oral thrush. If you notice white patches in your mouth, seek treatment from your doctor.

'If you notice white patches in your sore mouth, seek treatment from your doctor.'

- Dry mouth: In addition to sucking on ice chips and staying hydrated, you can also coat your mouth with butter or olive oil. Avoid dry foods and moisten foods with gravy and sauces. Use artificial saliva and lip balm. Avoid smoking, alcohol, and caffeine.

- Fingernail abnormalities and skin irritation: fingernails can crack, discolor, or develop lines associated with each cycle of chemotherapy. Avoid wearing anything on your nails including nail polish. Some chemotherapy drugs can cause generalized skin irritation on the feet and palms of the hands. This irritation can be treated with vitamins and by reducing the dose of those treatments. Skin irritation can also be caused if some of the chemotherapy drug accidentally drips or leaks onto the skin around the delivery port. This causes an immediate irritation and may take several weeks to calm. Ice, steroid injections under the affected skin, and anti-inflammatory creams can all provide relief. Notify your chemotherapy nurse immediately if this happens to reduce long-term damage.

'Notify your chemo-therapy nurse immediately if some of the chemo-therapy drug accidentally leaks onto your skin.'

- Sexual and reproductive issues: Like radiation, chemotherapy can also temporarily or permanently damage fertility. However, chemotherapy acts by interfering with a woman's hormones and can cause her to stop ovulating for up to 24 months after treatment or to enter early menopause. For men, the reproductive side effects vary with the chemotherapy drug that is used. In any case, never rely on chemotherapy or radiation as a form of birth control.

- Watery, gritty, sore eyes. Only a few chemotherapy drugs cause this side effect and it can be easily resolved by using eye rewetting drops.

- Diarrhea and constipation. This side effect can be caused by a few of the chemotherapy drugs and anti-nausea medication you may be prescribed. If your chemotherapy medications cause diarrhea, your doctors and nurses will warn you in advance and provide you with medication to deal with it. The key for both of these symptoms is to stay hydrated. Drink plenty of fluids and eat fresh fruit and other sources of fiber.

'Drink plenty of fluids and eat fresh fruit and other sources of fiber.'

What are the long-term side effects for radiation therapy and chemotherapy?

Some side effects take years to develop or notice. These will remain with you for the long-term.

Radiation therapy

Internal scarring is one of the most common long-term side effects of radiation therapy. Related to this is radiation damage to internal organs. Although these side effects are being reduced as newer methods of delivering radiation therapy are becoming more accurate, they are still a minor possibility. In addition, taste and salivary changes that occurred because of radiation treatment to the head or neck can become permanent. One other long-term effect of radiation therapy is that it can suppress the immune system making you more susceptible to infections and other cancers.

Chemotherapy

Long-term side effects caused by chemotherapy depend on the drugs used. Some of these include heart damage, kidney damage, lung damage, and nerve damage. Check with your doctor to find out the long-term side effects of the specific chemotherapy drugs you are using and to learn if there are certain symptoms for which you should be alert.

Are there any side effects I should tell my healthcare professional about?

If during treatment you experience any of the following side effects, you should contact your doctor straight away:

- A fever over 100.4°F (38°C). This could be a sign of a serious infection.

- You suddenly feel unwell.

- You become breathless.

- Severe headache and/or vision changes.

- Severe vomiting (unable to keep anything down).

- You feel faint or dizzy.

- Abdomenal pain.

- An allergic reaction, such as rash, swelling, or shortness of breath.

- Anxiety.

'Check with your doctor to find out the long-term side effects of the specific chemo-therapy drugs you are using.'

- Restlessness.

What can I do to help prevent side effects?

Preventing side effects depends on the side effect you are struggling with. Consider the following to help ease your symptoms:

'Pain, depression, anemia, and infections can all cause fatigue, so it is important to have a doctor evaluate you.'

- Fatigue: The key thing to remember is that if you are fatigued it does not mean that your cancer is getting worse, something is wrong with your treatment, or your cancer is coming back. Pain, depression, anemia, and infections can all cause fatigue, so it is important to have a doctor evaluate you even though this is a common symptom of treatment. All of these things can be corrected but only if you inform your medical team. You should also reduce the number of hours you work and cut back on your activities and social outings. Create breaks in your schedule so that you can take rests throughout the day especially around the times when you feel the most tired. Accept help when others offer to give it. Try gentle exercise, such as a 20-minute stroll. Even when you are feeling tired, mild exercise can pep you up. Listen to music or talk with friends to get your mind off the tiredness. Avoid temperature extremes. Eat right, and get plenty of fluids. Do not feel upset, worried, or guilty because of your tiredness. Do only the things you must do, and have others do the rest for you. Get plenty of sleep at night. Take a warm bath or drink a warm milky drink before bed, and if you are having trouble getting to sleep or staying asleep inform your doctor so he or she can help.

- Hair loss: Avoid using heated rollers and curling irons. Use shampoos and conditioners with fewer irritating chemicals, such as baby shampoos. Wash your hair a little less frequently. Avoid artificially coloring your hair or getting a perm. Switch to a shorter style. You can try scalp cooling, which involves wearing a chilled cap during treatments. However, you may need to change the cap if your treatment is long, and you may develop a headache from it. Generally, your hair will grow back a few months after your treatments are finished. Some people choose to wear scarves, wigs, or caps during treatment. Your insurance may cover a wig or at least pay for part of it.

'Your insurance may cover a wig or at least pay for part of it.'

- Nausea and vomiting: When your doctor gives you anti-nausea drugs take them as prescribed to prevent yourself from getting sick in the first place. Avoid foods that are spicy, fatty, or greasy. Nibble ginger crackers or sip ginger ale or ginger beer. Keep dry crackers by your bed to nibble on before getting up in the morning. Eat many little meals throughout the day and avoid big meals. Keep a window open to air strong smells. Purchase sea-bands (acupressure bands) at the pharmacist – some people find them helpful. Prepare foods without strong odors, such as cold salads, or have someone else prepare your meals for you. Avoid places that are known for having strong odors.

- Infections: Avoid people who are sick. Avoid crowded places. Avoid participating in sports where you need to share changing rooms and showers. Bath or shower daily, wash your hands after going to the toilet and before eating or handling food. Do not share items such as towels or soap with other family members or friends. Drink 8 cups of water per day. Brush your teeth with a soft brush twice a day and consult your doctor or nurse as to whether you should use mouthwash. Consider drinking a glass of cranberry juice or cranberry tea in the morning and evening every day or eating ½ cup of cranberries. Follow the orders of your doctors and nurses if they restrict your diet to protect your health.

'Drink 8 cups of water per day.'

- Sexual and reproductive issues: radiation and chemotherapy can temporarily or permanently damage fertility. In addition, women or men having radiation therapy on their sexual organs may find sex to be painful due to scarring, or they may become impotent. Talk with your doctor about your treatment and any reproductive risks associated with it. See if there are alternatives that will not cause infertility or reproductive problems. Consider storing your sperm or eggs before you begin treatment, and discuss this option with your doctor. Sometimes you may have to wait up to a year after treatment to prevent major birth defects before you attempt to become pregnant. Your doctor can help you plan appropriately.

- Skin irritation: avoid shaving the area that has become irritated. Use baby soap or mild unperfumed soap to wash in lukewarm water and pat the area dry. Only use the lotions, deodorants, and perfumes that your radiation care team has told you to use. Protect your skin from sunlight by keeping it covered and using a sunscreen rated SPF 15 or higher (even under clothing). Keep skin well-covered and protected from temperature extremes. Avoid swimming or talk to your doctor about what additional care (such as rinsing thoroughly and applying an aqueous cream afterward) you will need.

- Joint stiffness or muscle pain: develop a regular plan of exercise for the area where you usually get the pain. If the pain becomes troublesome, your doctor may refer you to a physiologist.

How do I keep a positive outlook while having side effects?

'The enemy may get in a blow or two here with tiredness, nausea, or skin irritation, but you are taking it down several notches with each treatment.'

If your treatments are helping destroy or stop your cancer, remember that you are fighting a war against it. The enemy may get in a blow or two here with tiredness, nausea, or skin irritation, but you are taking it down several notches with each treatment.

If your treatments help to reduce other effects from the cancer, keep in mind that your side effects are not as bothersome as what the original cancer effects were.

It is always good to create a journal of your thoughts and feelings, especially when you can share that journal with others. Do not just write it and forget it. Return to past entries and see how you felt and how you came through it. Compare how you felt then with how you are feeling now. If you are just beginning your journal, share it with others and get their feedback about it.

'A good way to deal with side effects is to join a support group.'

Most people find fatigue to be the most worrisome side effect even though it is also the most common. Talking it and other symptoms over with your doctor will help you determine if what you are feeling is normal. You should try to maintain some level of activity because too much rest can make you even more tired. If you begin to become so tired that you lose interest in things, let your doctor know. There are many treatments available to relieve this condition. Living with a constant feeling of tiredness will make even the most cheery person sad, so the sooner you can resolve this side effect, the better for you and your well-being.

Finally, a good way to deal with side effects is to join a support group. When others have gone through what you are experiencing, it can create a feeling of companionship. Trying to do something alone is always more difficult than trying to do it with others. Support groups can introduce you to people who have already been through what your are going through, people who are going through problems at the same time as you, and people who are just beginning their journey who want your advice and help for dealing with things you have already dealt with.

Summing Up

- Common side effects for radiation therapy are: fatigue; localized hair loss; skin burns, blisters, pain, peeling, or irritation; lowered blood counts; joint stiffness or muscle aches; and sexual and reproductive issues. Other side effects depend on what part of your body is receiving the radiation.

- Common side effects of chemotherapy are: fatigue; hair loss; lowered blood counts; nausea and vomiting; sore mouth; dry mouth; fingernail abnormalities and skin irritation; sexual and reproductive issues; watery, gritty, sore eyes; and diarrhea and constipation.

The long-term side effects of chemo-therapy depend on which drug(s) you are taking.

- The most common long-term side effect with radiation therapy is internal scarring. The long-term side effects of chemotherapy depend on which drug(s) you are taking.

- If you show signs of an infection, signs of an allergic reaction, suddenly feel unwell, are unable to control your vomiting, have a severe headache, have a severe stomach ache, have signs of anxiety or restlessness, or you feel dizzy, breathless, or faint, contact your doctor right away.

- There are many steps you can take to prevent or alleviate side effects. The first step you should always take is to talk with your doctor about them.

- Joining a support group can help keep your spirits high and make dealing with side effects easier.

'There are many steps you can take to prevent or alleviate side effects. The first step you should always take is to talk with your doctor about them.'

Chapter Five
How Can I Help My Friend or Family Member During Treatments?

What not to say.

There are many ways that people deal with the shock of finding out that a loved one has cancer. However, typically the first words that come out of your mouth are not well thought out words of wisdom. For some people, the first thing that comes to mind is death and other people they have known who died from cancer. When a person is diagnosed with cancer, they do not need to hear about dying. Not only is it likely that they will live, but such a depressing topic does nothing to boost his or her mood.

In the same way, do not feel like you should tell the person how badly you feel for them. This is similar to saying that they do not have a chance. Bob Perry has had prostate cancer for seven years. When he was first diagnosed, he was told he would only live one year. He states, 'I don't' want anyone feeling sorry for me. I don't feel sorry for me. There are a lot of people that are worse off than I am.'

'I don't' want anyone feeling sorry for me. I don't feel sorry for me. There are a lot of people that are worse off than I am.' - Bob

On the other hand, another verbal error is listing all the people you know that *are* worse off. While the person newly diagnosed with cancer does not want to be told they will soon die, they also do not want to be told how grateful they should be that it is not worse.

It is inappropriate to tell a cancer patient "treatments are easy" or "look on the positive side." These statements hurt more than help. Chances are good that treatments will be hard and you will make the patient more depressed and upset about going through it. They will blame themselves when things are tough. Cancer is a bad diagnosis. Although outcomes are more positive than in previous decades, the treatments are difficult to go through.

'Cancer is a bad diagnosis. Although outcomes are more positive than in previous decades, the treatments are difficult to go through.'

Sometimes people respond in a way that blames the person for getting cancer. There are many factors that come together to create cancer. Some can be controlled, but many cannot. Even if a person has had risky behaviors, he or she cannot go back in time and stop them. Adding to guilt the patient is already feeling is not helpful.

Equally bad is the response that makes light of the fact a person has cancer or attempts a joke about it. Neither of these is appropriate. If your friend wants to joke about his or her situation, by all means encourage the humor. However, you should not make jokes about it.

No matter how curious you are about some private aspect of cancer treatment, do not ask your friend or family member about it. If you are that curious, you can either go to the library, use the Internet to find the answer yourself, or you can ask your own doctor about it. There are some things no one wants other people to know about, and they should not be brought up in any polite conversation. In addition, there are certain questions you would never ask healthy individuals – such as, "Are you impotent?" "Are you going bald?" – It is equally rude to ask these questions to cancer patients.

Your friend's/family member's cancer is not about you or the patient's spouse or anyone related to the patient or anyone the patient knows. When you switch the topic abruptly to how the diagnosis is affecting others around him or her, it feels as if you have already dismissed any feelings the patient has. Sometimes previous cancer patients are the worst at this when they say something like, 'I know how you feel.' Although subtle, this switches the conversation away from the newly diagnosed patient to the one who has 'been there before.'

'Sometimes, it is best to just offer support.'

Sometimes, it is best to just offer support. Phrases like, 'I don't know what to say,' 'How are you doing, today?' 'What can I do to help,' or even simply, 'I am sorry to hear that.' Sometimes, no matter what you say, there may be a pause, or the person with cancer may read too much into what is said or not said. Keep in mind that this is an emotional time. Brief communication that is not overly positive, overly negative, overly self-centered, or overly rude is best.

Your friend or family member is going to have many choices to make about treatment. If he or she asks, you should help him or her research the options, but do not tell the patient what they should do. If they are willing to tell you what they are struggling with, you should be willing to listen without giving advice. If a cancer patient wants your opinion about treatment options, he or she will ask you directly.

Finally, there are many tough and difficult topics related to cancer that may make you uncomfortable to hear, but these may be the things the patient wants to talk about with you. If the patient brings up a topic that makes you uncomfortable, do you best to struggle through talking about it instead of trying to sweep it under the rug. Just talking about it can remove a giant weight from the person's shoulders. Take your time and think through your answers before responding.

'Although you should help him or her research the options, do not tell the patient what they should do.'

Ways to support.

Since the biggest, most common side effect of treatment is fatigue, the biggest help and support that you can give is to step up to the plate and do chores or errands for the patient. Helping around the house, bringing groceries, cooking, watching children, and walking pets are all ways to become physically involved in supporting your friend. Always offer to do something, and be specific in what you are offering. Never just leave the situation open ended by saying something like 'Call me if you need me.'

There are also emotional aspects to consider. Sometimes calling to talk – and then allowing your friend to do the talking– is very helpful. Going with him or her to the doctor's office and helping the patient take notes can be just as valuable. So can doing research for them and bringing them gifts that will help. Offer to help screen calls and to answer questions other people may have.

Visit your friend in the hospital and go with them for treatments to keep them company. Try to make time out of your day. Frequently, people tend to flit into a hospital room for ten minutes and say, 'Hi' and then flit away. In this case, it feels like you are only there out of duty instead of showing true compassion.

You may also volunteer to be the contact person for others. You could set up a website, e-newsletter, or blog that updates other friends and family members of the patient's needs and condition. If you are asked or volunteer to do this job, remember to be discrete.

'You could start a meal drive and arrange for others to donate meals on different days.'

If you work with the patient, volunteer to be in charge of a sick-day bank, if your employer allows this. This is where others can donate sick days for the patient to use. There are websites that allow you to help raise funds for the patient and his or her family – managing one of these will be greatly appreciated. Or, you could start a meal drive and arrange for others to donate meals on different days.

Sometimes you may have valuable specialized skills that you would like to donate. Volunteering to file insurance claims will take a weight off the patient's shoulders if you have skills in this area. Offering free legal services, if that is your expertise, will also be a relief to those who may want to write or adjust documents such as a power of attorney or living will.

Whatever you decide to do, just keep trying. Understand that this can be an emotional time for the patient, and he or she may not always respond in the way you expect. If you make a mistake when doing or saying something, just say you are sorry and move forward. The worst thing you can do is give up, or stop interacting with your friend or family member. Gifts and hugs are important, too.

Cheering up a sad friend or family member.

'Sit with them and hold their hand.'

As stated earlier, telling your friend or family member to cheer up, telling them they could be worse off, or trying to make a joke about their condition is not appropriate. Listening is appropriate and important. Bring them gifts that will help them through the times they are tired. Bring gifts that will keep them occupied during the wait while undergoing treatments in the hospital. The best gifts are books written by people who have survived cancer. Or, give the gift of yourself - sit with them and hold their hand.

Obviously, you should think about your gift before you give it, but most gifts will be well received. Consider unscented personal care items, recordings of favorite shows, light books, magazines, a list of websites related to the person's hobbies, socks, or something hand made. Just remember to call and ask when is a good time to come if you are delivering your gift personally.

You can also invite the patient to go with you to the movies, shopping, the park, or anywhere fun. Yes, there may be times when the patient is tired, but frequently these times come in cycles. You can always reschedule, and sometimes just the thought of being invited is enough to cheer them. You can also find ways to bring movies or a dinner home to them.

Chances are good your friend or family member will experience times of depression while he or she is going through treatments and fatigued. However, if the depression becomes great, you should try to go with your friend to the doctor and make the healthcare provider aware of it. Whenever someone talks about giving up or killing himself or herself, take note. If they begin to give away things they value, it is time to help them get help. Make them understand that they do not have to feel negative. Their doctor can help them with it.

'My husband took care of me – he fixed food and did not nag me even though I didn't eat much.'

- Shirley

Helping when energy is low.

Many cancer patients rely upon their spouse or partner to help them through their roughest times of feeling tired. Frequently they refer to going through cancer successfully as a "partnership." For example, Shirley Cowham, who had breast cancer and has been cancer free for 12 years states, "My husband took care of me – he fixed food and did not nag me even though I didn't eat much. He gave me support." She stated that she would lie on the couch for eight days after her chemotherapy and then have just enough energy to go for a drive with her husband on the ninth day. After that, she would read about six library books. By the time she finished she would just have gotten her energy back.

You can be a supporting partner as well. You can offer to take your friend or family member for a drive on the day when they begin to get their energy back, and you can bring them books to read, or yarn to knit, or anything else that might distract them from their tiredness.

'Even when energy is low, friends and family can find ways of encouraging and helping that go above and beyond the normal.'

However, recognize when you are asking too much. Bob states he felt frustrated when his friends asked him to do things that he just could not do. If your friend or family member is constantly telling you he or she cannot go golfing or eat the spicy food you brought, accept this and bring a ginger ale next time and a favorite movie.

Even when energy is low, friends and family can find ways of encouraging and helping that go above and beyond the normal. For example, if the patient had a quilt he or she wanted to make, friends and family can come together to finish it. If the patient normally plants a garden, but is feeling too tired during planting or harvest time, friends and family can come together to do it instead. Having everyone contribute stories of how the patient has helped others or of good times they had together and creating a book is another way of cheering a patient with low energy.

Learning more about your friend or family member's condition.

By reading this book, you have already taken a step in learning more about what your friend or family member is going through. Friends can be a great support and a great source of information. Do research and share what you learn. When you learn more, you show you are actively interested in your friend or family member and his or her treatment and recovery.

By attending doctor's visits, you can not only learn more about your friend's/family member's condition, but you can also help to record this information so that he or she has a resource to turn to if the anxiety and stress wipes the information from their memory.

Getting support for yourself.

Although watching someone go through cancer is not as difficult as actually going through it yourself, it is important to take care of yourself. Plan your days so that you get enough sleep, and eat meals regularly even if you do not feel like it.

You should also find your own source of support. There are many support groups for friends, family members, and caregivers of cancer patients. Do not hesitate to join one. You may even be able to attend with the person who is going through cancer.

'There are many support groups for friends, family members, and caregivers of cancer patients.'

Summing Up

- If you do not know what to say, tell the person just that. Do not allow the first words you speak to come out without thinking of all the implications they may have.

- Fatigue support and taking care of daily chores may be one of the most important physical things you can do for your friend, but emotional support is equally important.

- Something as simple as taking an hour out of your day to sit and hold your friend's hand at the hospital can go a long way to cheering him or her.

- Learn to recognize when your friend or family member's energy is the lowest and allow them the time to rest. If they constantly refuse the activities your offer, begin offering activities that require less energy.

- Do your own research and show what you learn to your friend or family member.

- Do not forget to take care of yourself. You should get enough sleep and food and emotional support. You can find support groups for friends, family members and caregivers throughout the US.

'Learn to recognize when your friend or family member's energy is the lowest and allow them the time to rest.'

Chapter Six
How Do I Reduce My Risk for a Relapse?

See your healthcare professional regularly.

The earlier you can catch cancer, or the earlier you can catch a relapse of cancer, the better your chances are of surviving it. Once a person has had cancer, their chances of getting it again increase. This is why you need to attend regular check-ups with your family physician and any other specialists as they are scheduled.

In addition, one cancer patient states 'I encourage anyone over 40 years old to get the screening.' If screenings are recommended or available, do not hesitate to continue having them. Screenings are not only used to show you if you have cancer, but also used to show you that you do not have it.

If your cancer returns, it could be the same kind or a different kind of cancer. Making sure that you are being screened for all the recommended types of cancer is a way to stay healthy and relieve anxiety.

'The earlier you can catch cancer, or the earlier you can catch a relapse of cancer, the better your chances are of surviving it.'

Do not ignore changes in your body.

Self-screening is another important way to be on your guard against a relapse. In addition to performing self-checks for breast or testicular cancer, you can notice signals your body may be sending to you. Self-screening allows you to take your survival into your own hands. As Larry, a cancer patient with multiple myeloma stated, 'Originally, I was given six months to live. Now I find that since I have had ten years, I would like ten more.'

'Originally, I was given six months to live. Now I find that since I have had ten years, I would like ten more.'

-Larry

Do not ignore it if blood appears in your stool or urine. Do not ignore lumps. When you feel sick, talk with your doctor about your symptoms. Do not ignore them.

At the same time, you do not have to be paranoid. That lump you see that looks like an abnormal mole may turn out to be benign. Do you need to have it checked? Yes. Do you need to take out an extra life insurance policy? No. Caution will keep you alive. Paranoia will drive you to an early grave.

Eat healthy.

It is important to have healthy options in your home that are easy to prepare and will provide you with the things your body needs. Increase the amount of leafy green vegetables and fiber that you eat. Try to eat at least one cup of fruit and one cup of vegetables each day. Get appropriate amounts of calcium, vitamin D, and protein.

Sometimes cancer treatments can cause you to lose your taste for certain foods. You can try eating new foods or you can drink shakes when you do not feel like anything else. Although you should work on getting your appetite back so you can maintain your strength, it is okay to rebuild it slowly. Also, there may have been some foods that your doctor asked you to stop eating while you were undergoing treatments. Ask him or her when you are able to eat them again.

You should also be sure to drink plenty of liquids. Fluids not only help to keep your body in balance, but they also allow you to clean it from the inside out.

Wash fruits and vegetables well before you eat them in order to remove any pesticide residue. Many pesticides and herbicides contain chemicals that cause cancer. Another good option is to switch to organic foods. Organic foods are grown without these chemicals.

'You can try eating new foods or you can drink shakes when you do not feel like anything else.'

Stop smoking.

Smoking increases your chances of dying from cancer by 30%. If you smoke, it should be at the top of you list to quit. Many insurance policies cover the cost of approved programs that help you quit smoking. Even state Medicaid programs are expanding to cover these costs because of the health benefits.

In addition, you should avoid secondhand smoke. Secondhand smoke causes around 3,400 lung cancer deaths in the U.S. alone each year.

Secondhand smoke is especially dangerous to children.

Reduce the amount of alcohol you drink.

Drinking more than 1 serving of alcohol each day increases your risk for several types of cancer. One serving of alcohol is 1.5 ounces (1 shot) of hard liquor, 8 ounces of wine, or 12 ounces of beer.

'Drinking more than 1 serving of alcohol each day increases your risk for several types of cancer.'

The younger a person begins to use alcohol heavily, the more the person increases their risks. If a person has five or more servings of alcohol per day, they are considered a heavy user.

If you would like to reduce your alcohol consumption but are finding it difficult to do so, there are programs available to help you. Your doctor can give you a referral if you need one.

Avoid tanning – indoor and outdoor.

It is best to avoid tanning beds. People who use tanning beds before the age of 35 increase their chances of getting skin cancer by 75%.

Tanning outdoors is also risky. Although 15 minutes in the sun helps your body produce vitamin D (which can reduce your risk of some cancers), spending more than an hour outside in direct sunlight without protection is a risk factor for skin cancer. It is best to seek shade. If you must be in direct sunlight wear a wide-brimmed hat that shades your face and neck (not a baseball cap). You should also wear clothing that covers your body, such as pants and long sleeved shirts, if you plan to spend extended periods of time in the sun.

Sunscreens that are labeled "broad spectrum" and have an SPF (sun protection factor) of 15 or higher can protect you from skin cancer. Apply sunscreens generously and frequently (at least as often as recommended on the labels). Always reapply after excessive sweating or swimming. Getting as few as five blistering sunburns can double your chances of getting skin cancer.

Hormone replacement therapy.

Hormone replacement therapy increases the chances of developing cancer again by 300%. It is important to discuss the risks and benefits of any hormone therapy, including hormonal birth control pills, with your doctor before beginning it.

Other things to avoid.

Some things are currently being researched because of their potential cancer risks. In addition, your doctor may recommend that you avoid things that are specific risks to redeveloping your type of cancer. The following is an incomplete list of potential cancer risk factors:

- Heat packs

- Raw or undercooked foods

- Red meat (beef, pork, lamb)

- Processed meats (hot dogs, sausage, bacon, cold cuts)

'Hormone replacement therapy increases the chances of developing cancer again by 300%.'

- Raw potatoes

- Saturated fats

- Charred meat

- Excessive salt

- Fried foods

- Junk foods

- Massage (especially at the tumor site)

Exercise.

Regular exercise helps to fight off depression, gives you more energy, reduces your risk of blood clots, takes your mind off things, and can improve your appetite. It enhances your immune system, helps you sleep better, regulates blood sugar, strengthens your bones and helps control your weight.

These benefits are all in addition to the fact that it fights obesity (another cancer risk factor) and is good for your body in general. It should not be surprising that research has shown exercise to decrease your chance of initially getting cancer and the chances it will return.

You do not have to run a marathon to get exercise even if you did this kind of strenuous activity before you had cancer. Start by walking around the park. You can also climb stairs, garden, ride a bike or swim. Any activity is good for you.

'Regular exercise helps to fight off depression, gives you more energy, reduces your risk of blood clots, takes your mind off things, and can improve your appetite.'

Always talk with your doctor before beginning any exercise program, but you can also talk to your doctor about a more structured exercise routine if you are interested in one. There are also many community exercise programs available from less intense ones, such as yoga, to more intense ones, such as water aerobics, at your local Y or community center. It is recommended that you exercise for a cumulative total of 2-½ hours of moderate exercise or 1-¼ hours of intense exercise each week.

'Continue to keep your body hydrated by drinking plenty of water.'

In addition to exercise that gets you moving, you should also work on muscle strength. You can do this by lifting small weights or even cans. Balance a stack of books on your legs and move them slightly up and down. Or work against gravity with exercises like push-ups and pull-ups.

Summing Up

- Continue seeing your doctor as frequently as recommended, and be sure to ask questions about any abnormalities even when your cancer is in remission.

- Self-checks for breast cancer or testicular cancer a quick easy reassurances you can do yourself. Do not ignore the signals your body may be sending you.

- Eat a well-balanced diet. If you have lost your taste for foods, try new ones or drink shakes. Continue to keep your body hydrated by drinking plenty of water.

- Quitting smoking is one of the most beneficial things a person can do to prevent cancer and its recurrence. Reducing secondhand smoke exposure also reduces cancer risks.

- Reducing the amount of alcohol you consume to one serving or less per day also reduces your cancer risk.

'Avoid indoor tanning beds, and protect yourself if you must be out in the sun for more than 1 hour.'

- Avoid indoor tanning beds, and protect yourself if you must be out in the sun for more than 1 hour. If you use sunscreen as a part of your sun protection, apply it generously and frequently.

- There are many things that may increase your chances of cancer. Some currently have minimal or inconclusive research relating them to cancer, but even a small increase in risk should be avoided. Your doctor will have a complete list of things to avoid that are specific to your cancer.

- Speak with your doctor about developing a regular exercise program. You can exercise passively by going on walks and lifting cans at home, or you can take an active part in developing an official exercise routine.

Chapter Seven
Resuming Your Life After Radiation and Chemotherapy

Expect setbacks. Push through plateaus.

Almost everyone recovering from cancer will have setbacks. These are normal. It is important, however, for you to expect them and prepare yourself mentally for them. Never blame yourself for setbacks, and keep in mind that most of them can be treated. Setbacks do not mean that you will never recover.

The best way to deal with setbacks is to make short-term and long-term goals for both your physical and emotional healing. Choose what you most want to accomplish and consider what things may keep you from accomplishing it. Keep checking your goals and adjust them as needed – especially when you experience a setback.

Equally as frustrating are plateaus where you are not sliding backward but do not seem to be moving forward either. If you experience a plateau, where it seems you have not made

'Never blame yourself for setbacks, and keep in mind that most of them can be treated.'

progress for a month or more, you need to make an appointment to discuss it with your doctor.

There are times when our bodies need a special boost or when the doctor might be able to give us new insight into why we are not moving forward. Discussing your plateau or setback with him or her will help you get past it.

Exercise.

Developing an exercise routine not only helps prevent cancer, but also improves recovery. Introducing a doctor approved exercise routine as one of your new daily habits will improve your mood and your overall outlook. It will also help you track your improvement.

'Developing an exercise routine not only helps prevent cancer, but also improves recovery.'

Losing your hair.

Although hair that was lost from chemotherapy will grow back, hair lost from radiation therapy might not. It can be exceptionally difficult to get over your cancer treatment when your hair is not growing back. If this is the case, you may want to consider purchasing a wig if you do not already have one.

Fighting fatigue.

Nearly two-thirds of all cancer patients experience fatigue. This can last even after treatments are finished. The best way to fight fatigue is to get enough rest, but that may be difficult.

To help get in the habit of resting, you need to create a routine – go to bed and get up as close to the same time as possible each day. Make sure you plan to get 8 hours of sleep each night. Do not do anything but sleep (and have sex) in your bedroom. Televisions, computers, and other objects that are backlit can all keep your brain artificially active longer than it wants to be.

Invest in black out curtains if outside light is affecting your quality of sleep. You should also arrange your bedroom so that other lights are not shining on you while you sleep or are trying to sleep.

Also, sleeping pills may help for a couple weeks, but long-term use of sleeping pills (longer than 4 weeks) can cause sleeping problems.

Other things you can avoid are:

- Avoid caffeine, nicotine, and alcohol for the 6 hours before your scheduled bedtime.

- Do not eat or drink a lot around your bedtime.

- Do not do exercise within 4 hours of your bedtime.

- Avoid watching television, playing video games, or working with anything that is backlit – especially in dark rooms within an hour of your bedtime.

- If possible, avoid naps during the day – especially in the later afternoon.

'Televisions, computers, and other objects that are backlit can all keep your brain artificially active longer than it wants to be.'

Things that help some people sleep:

- Drinking a cup of warm milk.

- Eating a turkey sandwich.

- Practicing relaxation techniques – such as imagery, deep breathing, etc.

- Taking a hot bath.

- Reading a book or listening to music for an hour before your bedtime.

'I am not saying that God heals everyone who has cancer, but He gives me the motivation and attitude to get through it.'

- Bob

Spirituality.

Many people turn to their religious faith to help them get through the tough times of cancer treatment. Prayer and meditation can provide hope and meaning when the rest of your life seems hopeless and your cancer seems meaningless. Faith can be a means of support during your treatments, and it can become especially important if you have finished your treatments and still have cancer.

Bob P. states the key to fighting depression is, 'Don't get down on yourself. You must tell yourself that it isn't the end and be determined that it isn't going to get you down. I am not saying that God heals everyone who has cancer, but he gives me the motivation and attitude to get through it.'

Allowing faith to be a part of your life in some way will help you fall back on something even when it seems like there is nothing left. It will give you peace and help you to deal with whatever is thrown at you. People who have some sort of spirituality tend to have better outcomes with cancer therapy, more positive thinking, and tend to be better at dealing with what is thrown at them.

Traveling.

During treatment, it can be very difficult to travel because traveling needs to be scheduled between breaks in treatment. In addition, you need to take your cancer file with you in case something happens while you are away. You will also need to stay within the US because of insurance availability, expensive health costs, and lack of facilities or treatments in other countries.

However, a month or two after you finish your treatment, you should be able to purchase travel insurance again and go where you would like. Be sure that you bring all of your medications in a long enough supply to account for difficulty with travel plans and returning late. Check to see if you will need any vaccinations before you go, and be sure to protect your skin from the sun.

'A month or two after you finish your treatment, you should be able to purchase travel insurance again and go where you would like.'

Having sex.

During cancer treatments, people can still have sex if their doctor approves, but several things change. First, people should use condoms. Getting pregnant while on chemotherapy or during radiation treatment is not recommended. The treatments can cause a spontaneous abortion if you do get pregnant, and if you manage to carry the baby full term, there are high risks for it to have severe genetic disorders. In addition, the hormones that run through a woman's body while she is pregnant can speed the spread and growth of any cancer. As a minor note, chemotherapy drugs can be released in semen and vaginal fluids and this can cause irritation to your partner if you do not prevent the exchange.

Second, during cancer treatments most patients are tired and lose interest in sex. People who are having trouble with sex – such as one partner would like to do it and the other would not – should talk to a doctor or counselor about their difficulties. This can help them come to a mutual agreement.

'Understand that having cancer treatments does not mean you will definitely be infertile afterward.'

Once cancer therapy has stopped, sex is fine. Understand that having cancer treatments does not mean you will definitely be infertile afterward. If you are not interested in having children, you should take measures to prevent that.

Sometimes the difficulties with having sex during cancer treatments can still remain. There can still be uneasiness and depression that are preventing partners from getting together. Women can experience dryness and need lubrication. They may develop a yeast infection, which should be treated by a doctor. Men may have problems getting or sustaining an erection. A doctor can also treat this.

In addition, the couple may need to get reacquainted before becoming sexually intimate. Here are some ideas for getting to know your spouse again:

- See a movie together.

- Go to a concert together.

- Have coffee together.

- Talk with each other about your feelings on issues you have been avoiding. Listen as much as you talk.

- Go on a bike ride together.

- Work on a puzzle together, or play a board game.

- Take a walk together, holding hands.

- Have a picnic together.

- Take a class and learn something new together.

- Go on a second honeymoon.

- Cook a meal together.

- Sit on the porch, watching the sunset and holding each other.

- Read to each other.

'If underlying depression is a reason couples are not having sex, they need to seek professional help.'

If underlying depression is a reason couples are not having sex, they need to seek professional help. Depression is a treatable disease.

If body image or the changes that the patient underwent during treatment are causing self-esteem issues, it can be helpful for the couple to talk about their feelings with each other and then seek professional help if that does not work to alleviate any concerns.

Having a baby.

Although there have only been smaller studies performed on women who have children after cancer treatments, the results show that there is no increased risk for a cancer relapse related to the pregnancy.

The main problem a couple may run into when trying to have a baby (aside from those mentioned that are related to sex) is that the patient may have lost fertility during treatment. For this reason, it is always recommended that the patient bank sperm or eggs before undergoing treatment to protect fertility afterward.

'I guess what I mean is that it will never be over, not for me. Everything is different now. Everything has changed.' - Briohne

The couple can always try natural methods first. If these do not work, the help of a fertility specialist can be enlisted. There are several methods that allow couples to have babies after being treated for cancer, but if none are successful, the couple can also choose to adopt children or babies.

Moving on.

Once you have cancer, it will always be there. Briohne Stokes survived breast cancer and writes in her play Powerfully Fragile: "I guess what I mean is that it will never be over, not for me. Everything is different now. Everything has changed."

Although you have survived cancer and cancer treatments, you may have created some habits during treatment that are no longer necessary.

You may also have formed good new habits that you should keep.

You will probably always have the cancer that was very much a part of your life in the back of your mind even when you conquer it. The key to moving forward with your life is not to allow it to consume you.

Summing Up

- During your recovery, expect setbacks and push through plateaus. Talk with your doctor when you have either to see if he or she can help you to overcome these.

- Exercise will speed your recovery and help prevent a cancer reoccurrence.

- Even if your hair has not grown back, you can still get on with your life. If scarves or headbands helped you get through before, it may be time to purchase a wig to help you move past the cancer and into the future.

- Developing good sleep routines will help you fight fatigue.

- Being spiritual helps people get through cancer treatments with a more positive outlook and higher success rate. It can also help people deal with life after cancer.

- Traveling is fine to do once you have finished your treatment. Take any

'Being spiritual helps people get through cancer treatments with a more positive outlook and higher success rate.'

medications you may be taking and protect your skin from exposure to the sun.

- Sex after chemotherapy is fine as long as you overcome any physical and emotional problems that may exist. During chemotherapy it is recommended the couple use condoms to protect each other from irritation and to keep from becoming pregnant.

- There are no studies linking having a baby after cancer treatment and a return of cancer. Having a baby may require fertility treatments or even adoption if the couple lost fertility during the radiation therapy or chemotherapy.

- Sometimes it can be difficult to move past having cancer. There will always be a cloud in the back of your mind that thinks about it. However, you do not have to let that interfere with living your life.

'There are no studies linking having a baby after cancer treatment and a return of cancer.'

Chapter Eight
FAQs

Can't people die from radiation?

Radiation is like any other medication: too much can kill you. However, this is why you have a team of doctors working together to give you the minimum amount of radiation you need to kill the cancer. Remember, the healthy cells in your body are stronger than the cancer cells. They can repair themselves quicker and more efficiently.

When I have radiation therapy will I become radioactive?

If you have external radiation therapy, the source of the radiation is located outside your body. Although the radiation will go through your body, your body cannot become a source that creates more radiation.

'Although the radiation will go through your body, your body cannot become a source that creates more radiation.'

When you have internal radiation therapy, a source that creates radiation is planted inside your body. Since this source emits radiation, you will be emitting radiation. However, your body does not become a source for radiation, and as the implanted material loses its radioactivity, you will emit less and less radiation. Generally, you must stay in the hospital until the source is emitting low enough levels of radiation that will not harm others. Before you are released, you will also be given guidelines to avoid exposing people who could even be harmed by lower levels of radiation.

If I start taking pain medication, will I become addicted to it?

As long as you follow the directions for taking pain medication as your doctor prescribes, and you inform all your doctors about all the drugs, supplements, and vitamins you are taking, you should not have trouble giving up the pain medication when you no longer need it. Your doctors will monitor you closely, and you can discuss any concerns you have with them.

'Although everyone experiences aches and pains that are part of life, constant severe pain from cancer can make it more difficult for you to maintain a positive attitude and heal.'

Although everyone experiences aches and pains that are part of life, constant severe pain from cancer can make it more difficult for you to maintain a positive attitude and heal.

Will my hair grow back?

People who lose their hair from radiation therapy may or may not have it grow back. It depends on the dose and length of exposure. People who lose their hair from chemotherapy will grow it back.

I am not feeling sick from my cancer. Can't I wait to decide?

The sooner cancer is treated, the better your chance to return quickly to a normal life. Waiting until you have symptoms caused by tumors can be too late. Cancer cells, by nature, grow and spread out-of-control. As they do this, they kill healthy cells that are doing their job. You may not develop symptoms until you have lost many healthy cells.

Regular screenings and self-examinations are recommended so cancer can be discovered before it has taken over your body. As soon as your doctor makes a cancer diagnosis, you should follow through with planning and treatments.

Cancer does not go away on its own. If it is large enough to be detected, that means that your immune system is not able to deal with it.

I heard that radiation therapy could cause more cancer. Is that true?

Exposure to radiation increases your chance for developing certain cancers. Research has shown that only about 5 in 1,000 people develop more cancer from radiation therapy treatments. This risk can increase or decrease depending on where in your body the tumor being treated is located. Keep in mind that having cancer once also increases your chance to get it again. Also remember that if your doctor prescribes radiation therapy, he or she has determined that the benefit of stopping the cancer you have far outweighs the risk of possibly developing cancer in the future from the treatments.

'Cancer does not go away on its own.'

I heard that chemotherapy could make your cancer worse. Is that true?

Chemotherapy usually kills cancer or stops its growth. However, it also damages healthy cells. Once a treatment is finished, these healthy cells work hard to repair themselves. While they are repairing themselves, they produce a protein that can help cancer cells nearby to grow and reproduce. Currently, only a few chemotherapy drugs have been tested with these results on only a few different cancers.

Although this recent research seems disturbing, it merely confirms why combination therapy and changing chemotherapy drugs is more effective. In addition, many people have taken chemotherapy and not had cancer return or had any future problems with cancer.

If you are concerned about how chemotherapy may act in your body, you can talk these concerns over with your healthcare provider.

'Radiation therapy can cause burns, but these are superficial and similar to sunburn.'

Won't radiation burn my skin (arm, breast, etc.) off?

Radiation therapy can cause burns, but these are superficial and similar to sunburn. Radiation therapy is carefully planned to avoid doing serious damage.

Did I get cancer because of something I did?

There are certain things, such as smoking that can increase your chances of getting cancer. However, most of the time, there is no known reason as to why a person developed cancer. Even if you had or have behaviors that increased your cancer risk, you should not blame yourself for the disease. Some people get cancer without practicing any risky behavior.

God wants me to have cancer so there is nothing I can do to get rid of it.

Even Paul, in Timothy 5:23, told Timothy to take a little wine as medicine for his frequent illnesses and stomach problems. Being ill does not mean God does not want you to seek treatment. It simply means we live in a fallen world.

I don't think my treatment is working because I don't feel sick from it.

Everybody responds to treatment in different ways. Although most people have some side effects that make them feel sick, some people do not have any.

Is cancer contagious?

'You cannot catch cancer from another person.'

You cannot catch cancer from another person. If your friend or family member gets cancer, you can continue sharing spaces with them and not worry that you will get it. Because people who live and work together are exposed to similar cancer risks and because cancer can be transferred through DNA in families, it may seem as if cancer is contagious.

You can, however, catch viruses, such as HPV, which cause cancer. Also, a person who has cancer generally has a weakened immune system. This means they can catch many diseases from you. You should stay away from people who are battling cancer if you become sick with any infection.

I finished chemotherapy last month. Why do I still feel badly?

It can take up to a year to feel back to normal. You just came through a major ordeal. You will need to give your body time to readjust.

If you experience setbacks or if you have a plateau where you are not making progress for more than a month, talk with your doctor and readjust your goals.

'Because radiation therapy and chemo-therapy both require exact doses to ensure they heal without doing further harm, it is important for doctors to be precise.'

Isn't there a natural cure that doctors haven't told us about?

There are many natural, complementary, or alternative treatments that relieve some of the side effects of chemotherapy and radiation. However, there is no scientific evidence showing that any of these methods can cure cancer.

There are certain chemotherapy drugs that were derived from plants. Radiation is also "natural" in the sense that it is found in nature. However, these treatments need to be regulated and prescribed by a doctor.

Plants and herbs contain varying amounts of the necessary chemicals depending on where they are grown and when they are harvested. Without going through FDA regulated purification and extraction processes, they cannot be given in specific doses. There is also no way to dose radiation found in nature or to pinpoint which part of your body receives it. Because radiation therapy and chemotherapy both require exact doses to ensure they heal without doing further harm, it is important for doctors to be precise.

In addition, some natural remedies that claim to be cures can actually hinder your healing process and interfere with the radiation and chemotherapy you are receiving. For this reason, please tell your medical team all the herbal supplements, vitamins, minerals, and alternative therapies you are using in addition to all your over-the counter and prescribed medications.

Doesn't surgery just spread cancer?

Surgery is one of the most important ways to get the cancer out of your body and stop it from spreading. Sometimes, the surgeons find more cancer than they expected, and sometimes the surgeons may not be able to remove all the cancer. This has lead to rumors that surgery makes it worse. However, removing the cancer does not cause it to grow any more than what it already was.

My sister survived breast cancer, and now, I have it. Why are my treatments different than hers?

When your medical team is planning your treatments, they take into account a number of different things. Your treatments are designed specifically for you. They will not necessarily be similar to the treatments that other people receive even if you have the same kind of cancer.

Your treatments are designed specifically for you. They will not necessarily be similar to the treatments that other people receive even if you have the same kind of cancer.

Will I glow in the dark after radiation?

No. People do not absorb enough radiation from radiation therapy to glow in the dark.

My doctor just prescribed chemotherapy. Does that mean I am going to die?

Chemotherapy is a treatment – not a death sentence. The treatments your doctor prescribes are based upon the type of cancer you have and where it is in your body. Chemotherapy is not a last resort treatment.

'There are many support groups throughout the US that are both national and local.'

In addition, cancer survival rates are increasing. Most of the people interviewed for this book are doing fine and were diagnosed with cancer for the first time more than five years ago. All of them underwent some sort of chemotherapy. Many of them also had radiation treatments.

Do antiperspirants cause cancer?

Currently, the best scientific research does not show a link between cancer and antiperspirants.

Where can I find a support group?

There are many support groups throughout the US that are both national and local. There are groups available for patients, caregivers, family members, and friends of people who have cancer. You can begin looking for one in the Help List section of this book. There, you will find organizations that offer support groups or that can direct you to one.

Summing Up

- You doctors and cancer team will carefully monitor the amount of radiation you receive in order for it to give you the most benefit with the least amount of damage.

- When you receive internal radiation therapy you will emit radiation until the source fades or is removed. You will not emit radiation after external radiation therapy.

- Treating pain is important. However, be sure to follow your doctor's instructions and let him or her know all the medications you take to prevent addictions.

'You should never wait to make a decision about treatment once cancer is diagnosed.'

- Although most chemotherapies cause you to lose your hair, it will grow back after treatment. If radiation is the source of your hair loss, whether or not it grows back is dependent upon the dose and length of time you had the radiation therapy.

- You should never wait to make a decision about treatment once cancer is diagnosed. The sooner cancer is treated, the better chance you have of recovering from it.

- Radiation therapy may slightly increase your chances of developing cancer. However, your doctor would only prescribe it if he felt the risks outweighed the benefits.

'You need to concentrate on what you can do to overcome the cancer instead of what you might have done to cause it.'

- Some studies in labs have shown that certain chemotherapy drugs have caused normal cells that are damaged to produce proteins that could help cancer cells that survived the treatments to grow and increase. People, however, have been using chemotherapy drugs for years and have had many successes.

- You may get a sunburn type burn from radiation therapy. However, doctors monitor doses to prevent permanent damage.

- Even if you had risky behaviors prior to developing cancer, you need to concentrate on what you can do to overcome the cancer instead of what you might have done to cause it.

- Having cancer does not mean that God wants you to have it.

- Some people do not get sick during treatment. Whether or not you are sick does not affect whether or not the treatments are working.

- Cancer is not contagious in that it can spread from one person who has cancer to another person. However, certain viruses increase your risk for developing cancer and these viruses can be spread.

- You may still feel sick for up to a year after you stop your cancer treatments. Talk to your doctor if you experience a setback or if you do not seem to be making progress.

- Some cancer treatments are from natural treatments, but there is no natural treatment that can cure cancer. Treatments need to be carefully monitored and doses measured accurately. Natural cures do not allow this.

- Surgery does not spread cancer.

- Different people have different treatment schedules even if they have the same type of cancer.

- You will not glow in the dark after receiving radiation therapy.

- Chemotherapy is not a last resort for cancer treatment. If your doctor prescribes it, that does not mean he or she thinks you are going to die.

- Antiperspirants have not been linked to cancer in research that is currently available.

- Support groups are located throughout the US You can begin looking for one in the Help List at the end of this book.

'Chemotherapy is not a last resort for cancer treatment. If your doctor prescribes it, that does not mean he or she thinks you are going to die.'

Glossary

Alkylating Agents

Chemotherapy drugs that work by targeting the DNA of cancer cells and that work by preventing the DNA from separating into two sets of directions when the cell tries to divide.

Angiogenesis

When a tumor builds new blood vessels inside it in order to keep itself alive.

Anti-emetics

Anti-sickness drugs.

Anthracyclines

Chemotherapy drugs developed from antibiotics that work by locking the two strands of DNA together and preventing them from separating to make copies of themselves.

Anti–metabolites

Chemotherapy drugs that work by embedding in the DNA and stopping it from completing a copy of itself.

Atom

The smallest piece of an element that still has all the properties of that element.

Benign Tumor

Tumor that is not life-threatening and does not spread to other parts of the body. These tumors are removed with surgery and generally do not come back. No other treatments are needed for them.

Biological Therapies

Cancer treatment that uses things that are naturally found in your body, such as hormones, to fight cancer.

Biopsy

Removing a piece of a tumor for closer examination by a pathologist.

Body Mass Index (BMI)

A way of measuring the amount of fat your body contains as a proportion of your overall weight. A doctor can help you determine this number.

Brachytherapy

Radiation therapy that uses radioactive solids implanted in or near the tumor to deliver radiation.

Cancer

Malignant tumors or the illness caused by malignant tumors.

Carcinoma

Malignant tumor that begins in skin tissue.

Cell

The smallest living part of your body.

Central Line

Thin plastic line implanted into a vein with the opening on your chest. Used for delivering chemotherapy drugs and taking blood for tests.

Cervical Cancer

Cancer that begins on a woman's cervix.

Chemotherapy

Cancer treatment that uses chemicals to destroy cancer cells.

Clinical Trials

Process of giving an experimental treatment to a limited number of patients in order to examine the safety and effectiveness of the treatment.

Colorectal Cancer

Cancer that begins in the intestines.

Combination Therapy

When two or more chemotherapy drugs are combined for treatment.

Computerized Tomography (CT) Scan:

Method that uses moving X-rays to generate 3-D images.

Conformal Radiation Therapy

Another name for intensity-modulated radiation therapy.

Connective Tissue

Tissue, such as bone, that provides support or connects and surrounds body parts and organs.

Continuous Infusion

Chemotherapy drugs that are delivered at home over many days and require regular check-ups to monitor.

Cytotoxic Medicine

A drug that is toxic or poisonous to cells that are dividing.

DNA

The directions inside your cell. Abbreviation for deoxyribonucleic acid.

Enzyme

Protein that is made by your cells and helps things move faster in your body often by bringing the needed chemicals closer together so they can combine easily.

Epithelial Tissue

Tissue, such as skin, that forms a thing protective layer around the body, internal cavities, organs and ducts.

External Radiation Therapy

Radiation therapy that uses a machine to focus radiation on specific parts of the body.

Fatigue

Tiredness.

Fraction

Part of the total amount of radiation a person is to receive during their radiation therapy. A fraction is one treatment.

General X-ray

An X-ray. A way of looking inside the body.

Glucose

A simple sugar that can be made radioactive and given to a patient to help make PET images.

Hepatitis

This is an inflamed liver caused by an infection. It can cause an overall feeling of sickness, jaundice, and loss of appetite.

High Dose Rate Brachytherapy

Thin tubes are inserted near the tumor with a higher dose of radiation that that provided by low dose rate brachytherapy. However, the tubes stay in for a shorter period of time.

HIV

Human immunodeficiency virus is a virus that attacks the immune system's T-cells and causes AIDS.

Hodgkin's lymphoma

Cancer that begins in the lymphatic system.

Hormonal Therapies

Cancer treatments that adjust the levels of hormones in your body to fight cancer cells.

Hormones

A chemical that the body makes to regulate itself. These work with DNA to turn on and shut off which directions are followed.

HPV

Human papillomavirus. An STD that can cause genital warts or be without symptoms. HPV can cause cervical cancer and may also cause cancer of the penis.

Hyperbaric Oxygen Therapy (HBOT)

Treatment that increases the amount of oxygen in the blood in order to combat some of the severe side effects of cancer treatment.

Hyperfractionated Radiation Therapy

Newly developed method of giving entire course of radiation therapy treatments over 12 days instead of several weeks.

Hypofractionated Radiation Therapy

Newly developed method of giving higher doses per treatment but fewer radiation therapy treatments to lower the overall amount of radiation a person receives.

Image-Guided Radiation Therapy (IGRT)

Uses imaging techniques in addition to the radiation therapy in order to confirm the tumor is being properly targeted.

Implant Brachytherapy

Also called low dose rate brachytherapy.

Implantable Port

Thin plastic line implanted into a vein with the opening under the skin (either on the chest or arm) that must be accessed by a special needle. Used for delivering chemotherapy drugs and taking blood for tests.

Intensity-Modulated Radiation Therapy (IMRT)

Uses radiation therapy beams to give a very precise dose of radiation and enables the beam to be shaped to conform precisely to the shape of the tumor, which reduces side effects.

Internal Radiotherapy

When a source of radiation is introduced into your body and placed in or near a tumor.

Intra-Operative Radiation

When radiation therapy is giving during the surgery to remove the tumor.

Intravenous Injection

An injection into a vein.

Laryngeal Cancer

Cancer that begins in the voice box.

Leukemia

Malignant tumor that begins in the blood.

Linear Energy Transfer (LET)

The rate at which the radiation used is depositing energy in the tissue.

Low Dose Rate Brachytherapy

When between 80 and 100 seeds containing a low dosage of radiation are implanted in or near the tumor.

Lumbar Puncture

When a small needle is inserted into your lower back in the space next to the spinal cord in order to deliver chemotherapy medications to your brain or spinal cord.

Lymphatic System

A system within the body for fighting disease that delivers lymphocytes to the bloodstream and removes debris and microorganisms.

Lymphocyte

Cell of the immune system that is responsible for getting rid of foreign material. It is one type of white blood cell.

Lymphoma

Malignant tumor that begins in the lymphatic system.

Magnetic Resonance Imaging (MRI)

Use of strong magnets to read signals sent by water in your body, which detects contrasts between soft tissues.

Malignant Tumor

Tumor that can spread to other parts of the body and be life-threatening. These tumors are the same as saying someone has cancer. They can destroy healthy cells and have four forms: carcinomas, leukemias, sarcomas, and lymphomas.

Mammogram

X-ray that is specialized for detecting breast cancer.

Mesothelioma

Malignant tumor that begins in the lining of a body cavity.

Metastasize

When a malignant tumor spreads to another part of the body and begins to grow.

Molecule

The smallest piece of something that can exist by itself. These are made of two or more atoms that have bonded together.

Myeloma

Cancer of blood plasma cells.

Non-Hodgkin's Lymphoma

A cancer of the lymphatic system that is different from Hodgkin's lymphoma.

Nuclear Medicine

Uses a small amount of radioactive material injected into the body to allow the doctor to assess how certain areas are functioning.

Esophageal Cancer

Cancer that begins in the throat.

Obesity

Having BMI or Body Mass Index of more than 30.0. Your doctor can help you find your BMI.

Oncologist

A doctor who specializes in treating cancer.

Oral Cancer

Cancer that begins in the mouth.

Ovarian Cancer

Cancer that begins in a woman's ovary.

Pancreatic Cancer

Cancer that begins in the pancreas.

Pathologist

A scientist who is skilled in learning the cause of disease and if a disease is present. They test body samples for cancer.

Peripherally Inserted Central Catheter (PICC) Line

Thin plastic line implanted into a vein usually with an opening on the arm. Used for delivering chemotherapy drugs and taking blood for tests.

Photodynamic Therapy (PDT)

Cancer treatment that uses light or lasers to destroy cancer cells.

Pinhole Surgery

Also called low dose rate brachytherapy.

Plant Alkaloids

Chemotherapy drugs developed from natural plants that are also known as spindle poisons.

Platinum Compounds

Chemotherapy drugs that bind the strands of DNA together and prevent them from making copies of themselves.

Positron Emission Tomography (PET) Scan

Uses a radioactive material, such as glucose, that is normally broken down by healthy cells. Since cancer cells use glucose differently, it allows doctors to see them. It is used in combination with a CT scan.

Prostate

A gland found only in men that produces a fluid to aid in reproduction.

Prostate Cancer

Cancer that begins in a man's prostrate.

Protein

Product made by cells from amino acids. They are necessary for life functions and structure.

Proton Beam Therapy (PBT)

Radiation therapy that uses a beam of protons in the same way traditional radiation is used.

Radiofrequency Ablation (RFA)

Cancer treatment that uses radio waves to heat and destroy cancer cells.

Radiosurgery

Also called intra-operative radiation.

Radiation therapy

Cancer treatment that uses high-energy rays to destroy cancer cells.

Sarcoma

Malignant tumor that begins in connective tissue.

Seed Implant Brachytherapy

Also called low dose rate brachytherapy.

Spindle Poisons

Chemotherapy drugs that destroy the inside structure of a cell and prevent it from dividing.

Stem Cell

An undifferentiated cell that is not cancerous and can become several different types of cells.

Stereotactic Radiation Therapy

Uses many radiation therapy beams to target the tumor from different angles, lowering the amount of radiation normal cells receive while delivering the same dose to cancer cells.

Sun Protection Factor (SPF)

The amount of protection your skin receives from sunscreen. An SPF of 15 or more is recommended in order to reduce your cancer risk.

Supportive Therapies

Therapies given to people in addition to cancer treatments to help reduce side effects.

Systematic Approach

A treatment that involves the entire body instead of a small portion of it.

Testicular Cancer

Cancer that begins in a man's testicle.

Tissue

A group of cells that have a similar function or form. There are four basic types of tissues: muscle, skin (epidermal), connective, and nerve.

Topoisomerase

An enzyme in each cell that helps DNA copy itself.

Topoisomerase Inhibitors

Chemotherapy drugs that clamp onto the enzymes that help to copy DNA and prevent them from working.

Total Body Irradiation (TBI)

Used for people receiving stem cell transplants and often combined with chemotherapy.

Treatment Plan

A plan developed by your healthcare professional team that best treats your cancer.

Tubulin

A specialized protein that gives cells structure and helps them to divide.

Tumor

A mass of cells with mixed-up directions. These cells do not die even when they are not functioning properly and keep dividing even when they are too crowded. These can be either benign or malignant.

Ultrasound

Uses sound waves to create pictures of muscles, fluid filled spaces, organs, and bone surfaces.

Undifferentiated

Without distinguished characteristics.

Uterine Cancer

Cancer that begins in a woman's womb.

Vaginal Cancer

Cancer that begins in a woman's vagina.

Volumetric Modulated Arc Therapy (VMAT)

Uses three-dimensional imaging techniques to help pinpoint the area being radiated.

Vulval Cancer

Cancer that begins in a woman's vulva.

Help List

American Cancer Society

250 Williams Street NW, Atlanta, GA, 30303

Tel: 1-800-227-2345

www.cancer.org

The American Cancer Society is a national organization devoted to getting rid of cancer. There are many regional and local offices located throughout the country to better serve people. They focus on research, advocacy, education, and service. They also offer several different social networks for cancer patients, caregivers, and the friends and family of cancer patients.

American Childhood Cancer Organization

P.O. Box 498, Kensington, MD, 20895-0498

Tel: 1- 855-858-2226

www.acco.org

Website designed for children who are cancer patients and their families. They offer a variety of information on advocacy, research, awareness, and even resources such as books.

Canadian Cancer Society

55 St. Clair Avenue West, Suite 300, Toronto, Ontario, Canada, M4V 2Y7

Tel: 416-961-7223 (in Canada)

E-mail: ccs@cancer.ca

www.cancer.ca

Helps Canadians find relevant cancer information based upon where they live in Canada. They are community-based on a national level and seek to enhance cancer patients' quality of life and eradicate cancer.

Cancer.Net

American Society of Clinical Oncology (ASCO), 2318 Mill Road, Suite 800, Alexandria, VA, 22314

Tel: 1-571-483-1780 or Toll free: 1-888-651-3038

E-mail: contactus@cancer.net

www.cancer.net

Cancer.net was created to provide cancer patients, their caregivers, friends, and family members with the best cancer information. Its mission is to give patients the information they need to make the best decisions and allow them to become partners with their doctors in their cancer treatment. They have a great informational page on managing the cost of cancer here: http://www.cancer.net/navigating-cancercare/videos/cancer-basics/navigating-challenges-managing-cost-your-cancer-care

Cancer Support Community

1050 17th Street, NW Suite 500, Washington, DC, 20036

Tel: 202-659-9709 or Toll-free: 1-888-793-9355

http://www.cancersupportcommunity.org/

The Wellness Community is an online resource for support. There are support groups for cancer patients, family, and friends.

CancerCare

275 Seventh Avenue, New York, NY, 10001

Tel: 1-800-813-HOPE (1-800-813-4673)

www.cancercare.org

CancerCare is a support service that provides support groups, education, counseling, financial assistance, and publications free of charge. It helps people deal with the financial, emotional, and practical challenges of cancer by connecting them with professional oncology social workers.

Cancer Symptoms

www.cancersymptoms.org

Cancer Symptoms is a resource that not only helps with early detection and prevention, but also with managing symptoms experienced during treatment.

Children's Treehouse Foundation

50 South Steele Street, Suite #810 Denver, CO, 80209

Tel: 1- 303-322-1202

www.childrenstreehousefdn.org

This foundation was established to help improve the mental health of children whose parents have been diagnosed with cancer.

Hope for Two

P.O. Box 253, Amherst, NY, 14226

Tel: 1-800-743-4471

www.pregnantwithcancer.org

Hope for Two is an organization for pregnant women who have cancer. It provides support, information, and hope from women who had cancer while pregnant and survived.

Healthcare Hospitality Network

P.O. Box 1439, Gresham, OR, 97030

Tel: 1-800-542-9730

www.hhnetwork.org

The Healthcare Hospitality Network provides free or reduced lodging to patients and their caregivers when they are away from home seeking medical treatment.

Look Good… Feel Better

P.O. Box 1439, Gresham, OR, 97030

Tel: 1-800-395-LOOK (1-800-395-5665)

www.lookgoodfeelbetter.org

This websites helps you look good during your treatment with beauty tips from professionals. Targeted toward women, but there are also programs for men and teens.

Macmillan Cancer Support

89 Albert Embankment, London, U.K. SE1 7UQ or P.O. Box 2058, Belfast, U.K. BT59EH

International Tel: 011-44-207-840-7840 or 011-44-300-100-0200
www.macmillan.org.uk

This is a British support site that provides free information and emotional support for people living with cancer, including cancer types, treatments and what to expect, as well as information about US cancer support groups and organizations.

Memorial Sloan-Kettering Cancer Center (Integrative Medicine)

1275 York Avenue, New York, NY, 10065

Tel: 1-212-639-2000

http://www.mskcc.org/cancer-care/integrative-medicine

This is a web page sponsored by a cancer hospital that shows the wide variety of supplemental, alternative medicine practices that can be used for cancer patients.

National Cancer Institute (NCI) at the National Institutes of Health (NIH)

9609 Medical Center Drive, Bethesda, MD, 20892-9760

Tel: 1-800-4-CANCER (1-800-422-6237)

www.cancer.org

NCI is the government's primary agency for cancer research and training. It supports a nationwide network of cancer centers and research laboratories as well as coordinating information between facilities.

National Caregivers Library

901 Moorefield Park Drive, Suite 100, Richmond, VA, 23236

Tel: 1-804-327-1111

http://www.caregiverslibrary.org

Comprehensive website filled with the things you need to know about being a caregiver and resources for caregivers.

National Center for Complementary and Alternative Medicine (NCCAM)

Tel: 1-888-644-6226

http://nccam.nih.gov

The National Center for Complementary and Alternative Medicine is an extensive resource devoted to collecting scientific research on the effectiveness of alternative and complementary medicine.

National Comprehensive Cancer Network (NCCN)

275 Commerce Drive, Suite 300, Fort Washington, PA, 19034

Tel: 215.690.0300

http://www.nccn.org

The National Comprehensive Cancer Network is a collaborative group of top cancer centers wanting to improve cancer care quality and effectiveness. Their website contains information on living with cancer and resources including access to payment assistance programs.

Needy Meds

NeedyMeds, Inc., P.O. Box 219, Gloucester, MA, 01931

Tel: 1-800-503-6897

http://www.needymeds.org

Prescription discount cards are advertised on here, but if you type in the name of your medication, you will be shown patient assistance program information where you can apply to get the meds at low- or no-cost.

Quackwatch, Inc.

www.qwackwatch.com

This is an interesting website that posts warnings about potential medical frauds and myths. It covers a wide variety of resources.

ReMission2

www.remission2.org

ReMission allows young cancer patients to fight cancer in a video game atmosphere. It helps put real-world strategies into the hands of the patients in a virtual atmosphere. It was designed to encourage young patients to adhere to their treatment plans while providing them with a better feeling of control and power over their cancer. These games are freely provided by the sponsors of Hope Lab.

Sisters Network Inc.

2922 Rosedale St., Houston, TX, 77004

Tel 1-713-781-0255 or 1-866-781-1808

E-mail: infonet@sistersnetworkinc.org

www.sistersnetworkinc.org

This charity was established to bring awareness about breast cancer to the African American community and draw attention to the devastating impact breast cancer has on them.

The Susan G. Komen Breast Cancer Foundation

5005 LBJ Freeway, Suite 250, Dallas, TX, 75244

Tel: 1-877- GO KOMEN (1-877-465-6636)

E-mail: helpline@komen.org

ww5.komen.org

This organization strives to end breast cancer worldwide through community health outreach, research, programs, and advocacy.

The Ulman Cancer Fund for Young Adults

921 E. Fort Ave., Suite 325, Baltimore, MD, 21230 or 6310 Stevens Forest Road, Suite 210, Columbia MD, 21046

Tel: 1-410-964-0202 Ext. 1 or 1-888-393-3863 Ext. 1

www.ulmanfund.org

This fund is dedicated to providing various support programs for young adults who have been diagnosed with cancer. It focuses on developing resources, including those that allow young patients to share their journey, sharing information, increasing awareness, and empowering cancer survivors.

References

Abel, E. K., Subramanian, S. K., (2008) After the Cure; The Untold Stories of Breast Cancer Survivors. New York University Press.

American Cancer Society [Online] Available from http://www.cancer.org/aboutus/sitemap/index [accessed 03 August 2013]

Brown, Z. K., Boatman, K. K., (2009) 100 Questions & Answers About Breast Cancer *Third Edition*. Jones and Bartlett Publishers.

Cancer Recovery Foundation [Online] Available from http://cancerrecovery.org.uk/index [accessed 03 August 2013]

Cancer Research US [Online] Available from http://www.cancerresearchuk.org/home/ [accessed 03 August 2013]

Cancer Survival Statistics [Online] Available from http://www.cancerresearchuk.org/cancer-info/cancerstats/survival/england-and-wales-cancer-survival-statistics [accessed 03 August 2013]

Cancer Trends Progress Report – 2011/2012 Update, National Cancer Institute, NIH, DHHS, Bethesda, MD, August 2012, [Online] Available from: http://progressreport.cancer.gov [accessed 17 November 2014]

Chemo 'undermines itself' through rogue response [Online] Available from:

http://www.bbc.co.uk/news/health-19111700
[accessed 03 August 2013]

Clinical Trials [Online] Available from
http://www.macmillan.org.uk/Cancerinformation/C
ancertreatment/Clinicaltrials/Clinicaltrials.aspx
[accessed 03 August 2013]

Clinical Trials [Online] Available from
http://www.royalmarsden.nhs.uk/diagnosis-
treatment/pages/clinical-trials.aspx [accessed 03
August 2013]

Cukier, D., Gingerelli, F., Markari-Judson, G.,
McMullough, V. E., (2005) Coping with
Chemotherapy and Radiation. McGraw-Hill.

Ellsworth, P., (2009) 100 Questions & Answers
About Prostate Cancer *Second Edition*. Jones and
Bartlett Publishers.

Flynn, M., Barr, N. V., (2010) The Pink Ribbon
Diet. Lifelong Books.

Goodhart, F., Atkins, L., (2013) The Cancer
Survivor's Companion; Practical Ways to Cope with
Your Feelings After Cancer. Little, Brown Book
Group (?).

Kalick, R. (2004) Cancer Etiquette. Lion Books
Publisher.

Keane, M., Chace, D., (1997) The What to Eat if
You Have Cancer Cookbook. Contemporary Books.

Macmillan Cancer Support [Online] Available from
http://www.macmillan.org.uk/Home.aspx
[accessed 03 August 2013]

Mayo Clinic Staff, (2012) The Mayo Clinic Breast Cancer Book. Good Books.

McKay, J., Schacher, T., (2009) The Chemotherapy Survival Guide *Third Edition*. Newharbringerpublications, inc.

More people 'are surviving cancer' [Online] Available from: http://www.bbc.co.uk/news/world-20624891 [accessed 03 August 2013]

National Cancer Institute [Online] Available from http://www.cancer.gov/ [accessed 03 August 2013]

Patient.co.uk [Online] Available from http://www.patient.co.uk/ [accessed 03 August 2013]

Pratt, S. G., Matthews, K., (2006) SuperFoods HealthStyle; Proven Strategies for Lifelong Health. HarperCollins Publishers.

Priestman, T. (2005) Coping with Chemotherapy. Ashford Colour Press.

The Royal Marsden [Online] Available from http://www.royalmarsden.nhs.uk/pages/home.asp x [accessed 03 August 2013]

Shaw, G. M., (2011) Having Children After Cancer. Celestial Arts Berkley.

Silver, J. K., (2006) After Cancer Treatment; Heal Faster, Better, Stronger. The John Hopkins University Press.

www.ingramcontent.com/pod-product-compliance
Lightning Source LLC
Chambersburg PA
CBHW051717170526
45167CB00002B/695